Practical Manual of
Biochemistry

Name ....

Year ....

Roll no. ....

College ....

Teacher's Signature ....

ADVISORY COMMITTEE

Dr Biswajit Das
Professor and Head, Department of Biochemistry
Rohilkhand Medical College, Bareilly, UP

Dr Sohil Takodara
Associate Professor, Department of Biochemistry
Geetanjali Medical College and Hospital, Udaipur, Rajasthan

Dr Anupama Basvraj Patne
Associate Professor, Department of Biochemistry
American International Institute of Medical Science
Udaipur, Rajasthan

Dr Biswajit Das
Professor and Head, Department of Biochemistry
Rohilkhand Medical College, Bareilly, UP

Dr Deepa Thadani
Professor and Head, Department of Biochemistry
JLN Medical College, Ajmer, Rajasthan

Dr Tariq Mahmood
Associate Professor and Head, Department of Biochemistry
SRMSIMS, Bareilly, UP

Dr Sanjay Bhatt
Associate Professor, Department of Biochemistry
SRMSIMS Bhojipura, Bareilly, UP

Dr Manoj Gupta
Assistant Professor, Department of Biochemistry
SRMSIMS Bhojipura Bareilly, UP

Dr Shalini Gupta
Professor and Head, Department of Biochemistry
Government Medical College, Bharatpur, Rajasthan

Dr Neeta Sahi
Associate Professor and Head, Department of Biochemistry
PMCH, Udaipur, Rajasthan

Dr Sumeru Samanta
Assistant Professor, Department of Biochemistry
Rohilkhand Medical College, Bareilly, UP

Dr Devajit Sarmah
Professor and Head, Department of Biochemistry
GMCH, Faizabad, UP

Dr Randeep Mukherjee
Assistant Professor, Department of Biochemistry
GMCH, Faizabad, UP

Dr Shrawan Kumar
Professor and Head, Department of Biochemistry
Pandit Deendayal Upadhayay Medical College
Churu Rajasthan

Dr Manish K Singh
Assistant Professor and Head, Department of Biochemistry
Government Medical College
Badaun, Rajasthan

Dr Dharmveer Yadav
Associate Professor, Department of Biochemistry
AIIMS, Jodhpur, Rajasthan

Dr Shuchi Goyal
Professor and Head, Department of Biochemistry
RNT Medical College, Udaipur, Rajasthan

Dr Kanchan Sonone
Associate Professor, Department of Biochemistry
Lokmaniya Tilak Medical College, Sion, Mumbai
Maharashtra

Dr Ravi Shankar Chaudhary
Assistant Professor, Department of Biochemistry
Geetanjali Medical College and Hospital, Udaipur
Rajasthan

Dr Vinay Gehlot
Senior Demonstrator, Department of Biochemistry
Geetanjali Medical College and Hospital, Udaipur
Rajasthan

Dr Prashant Hisalkar
Professor and Head, Department of Biochemistry
Government Medical College, Dungarpur, Rajasthan

Practical Manual of
Biochemistry

GG Kaushik MBBS, MD, PhD, DRIA, FISC
Senior Professor
Department of Biochemistry and
Additional Principal
Jawaharlal Nehru Medical College and Hospital
Ajmer, Rajasthan

Neha Sharma PhD
Associate Professor
Department of Biochemistry
Geetanjali Medical College and Hospital
Udaipur, Rajasthan

Sabira Dabeer MBBS, MD
Assistant Professor
Department of Biochemistry
Geetanjali Medical College and Hospital, Udaipur
Rajasthan

Ruchi Jindal BDS, MSc (medical)
Demonstrator
Department of Biochemistry
Geetanjali Medical College and Hospital
Udaipur, Rajasthan

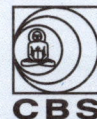

CBS

CBS Publishers & Distributors Pvt Ltd

New Delhi • Bengaluru • Chennai • Kochi • Kolkata • Mumbai
Bhopal • Bhubaneswar • Hyderabad • Jharkhand • Nagpur • Patna • Pune
• Uttarakhand • Dhaka (Bangladesh) • Kathmandu (Nepal)

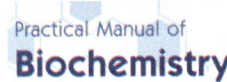

Practical Manual of

Biochemistry

ISBN: 978-93-89396-30-0

Published by Satish Kumar Jain and produced by Varun Jain for

CBS Publishers & Distributors Pvt Ltd

4819/XI Prahlad Street, 24 Ansari Road, Daryaganj, New Delhi 110 002, India.

Ph: 23289259, 23266861, 23266867   Website: www.cbspd.com

Fax: 011-23243014   e-mail: delhi@cbspd.com; cbspubs@airtelmail.in

Corporate Office: 204 FIE, Industrial Area, Patparganj, Delhi 110 092

Ph: 4934 4934   e-mail: publishing@cbspd.com; publicity@cbspd.com

Fax: 4934 4935

Branches

- **Bengaluru:** Seema House, 2975, 17th Cross, K.R. Road,
  Banasankari 2nd Stage, Bengaluru 560 070, Karnataka
  Ph: +91-80-26771678/79   Fax: +91-80-26771680   e-mail: bangalore@cbspd.com

- **Chennai:** 7, Subbaraya Street, Shenoy Nagar, Chennai 600 030, Tamil Nadu
  Ph: +91-44-26680620, 26681266   Fax: +91-44-42032115   e-mail: chennai@cbspd.com

- **Kochi:** 42/1325, 1326, Power House Road, Opposite KSEB Power House,
  Ernakulam 682 018, Kochi, Kerala
  Ph: +91-484-4059061-65   Fax: +91-484-4059065   e-mail: kochi@cbspd.com

- **Kolkata:** 6/B, Ground Floor, Rameswar Shaw Road, Kolkata-700 014, West Bengal
  Ph: +91-33-22891126, 22891127, 22891128   e-mail: kolkata@cbspd.com

- **Mumbai:** 83-C, Dr E Moses Road, Worli, Mumbai-400018, Maharashtra
  Ph: +91-22-24902340/41   Fax: +91-22-24902342   e-mail: mumbai@cbspd.com

Representatives

• Bhopal	0-8319310552	• Bhubaneswar	0-9911037372	• Hyderabad	0-9885175004
• Jharkhand	0-9811541605	• Nagpur	0-9421945513	• Patna	0-9334159340
• Pune	0-9623451994	• Uttarakhand	0-9716462459	• Dhaka (Bangladesh)	01912-003485
• Kathmandu (Nepal)	977-9818742655				

Printed At : Goyal Offset Works (P) Limited

Preface

The zeal to share our knowledge and experience has driven us to write this book. It has been written in simple language for easy understanding of basic concepts of practical biochemistry, taking into consideration various problems faced by healthcare professionals in biochemistry. The book caters the need of all the healthcare professionals.

Salient features of the book

- It covers the entire syllabus of medical biochemistry, core competency based.
- Includes flowcharts and diagrams for easy understanding.
- Presence of color pictures for clear visualization and understanding.
- Formation of working reagents has also been described in each chapter along with experiments.
- It includes viva voce, biomedical waste segregations and disposal.

This is our first edition and in spite of all precautions inadvertent mistakes are likely to happen. We would appreciate if the same is bought to our notice, so we can improve our self in next edition. We hope this book will be helpful to the students.

"A person who never made a mistake never tried anything new"—Albert Einstein

GG Kaushik
Neha Sharma
Sabira Dabeer
Ruchi Jindal

Acknowledgments

First and foremost, we would like to thank God Almighty for his kind blessings on us. Our sincere thanks and gratitude to Dr FS Mehta, Dean, Geetanjali Medical College, and our colleagues of Geetanjali Medical College and Hospital, Udaipur. Our special thanks to Ankita Sharma, Senior Demonstrator and the entire Department of Biochemistry of JLN Medical College, Ajmer, Rajasthan.

Our humble and sincere thanks to Mrs Ritu Chawala, Mr Dinesh S Dheek and CBC Publishers & Distributors for their trust on us.

We would also like to acknowledge the support of technical staff and postgraduate students for their help. We wish them good luck in their future endeavour.

Last but not the least, our thanks to our families, we cannot repay the constant support and encouragement from them.

GG Kaushik
Neha Sharma
Sabira Dabeer
Ruchi Jindal

Contents

Section 4
Miscellaneous

Index of Competencies

As per Medical Council of India: Competency Based Undergraduate Curriculum for the Indian Medical Graduate

INTRODUCTION TO PRACTICAL LABORATORY

Equipment and Instruments Used in Biochemistry Laboratory

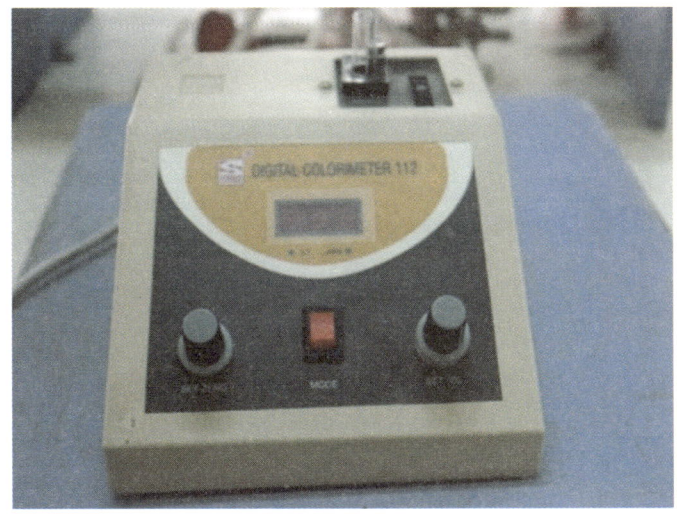

Colorimeter

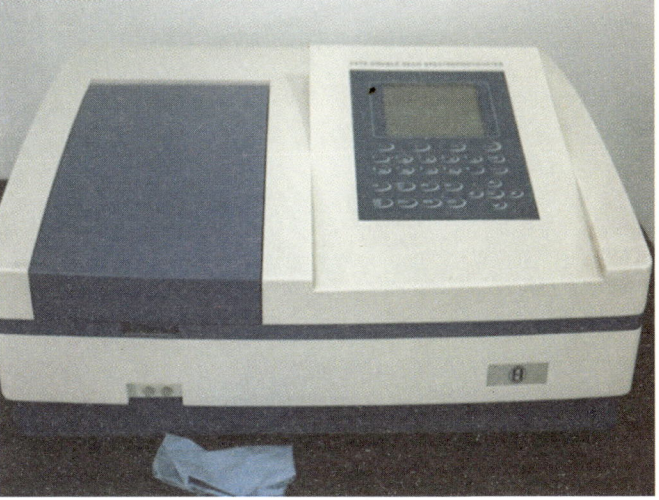

Spectrophotometer

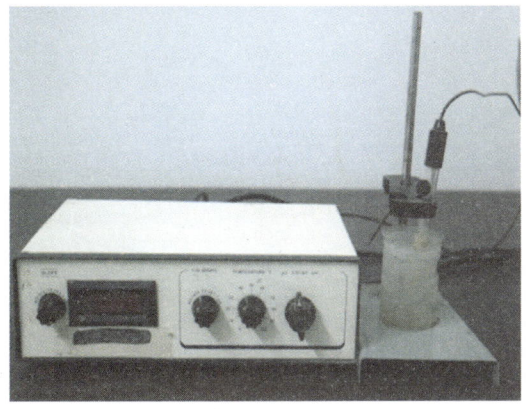

pH meter

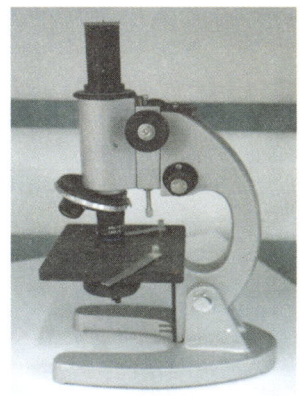

Microscope

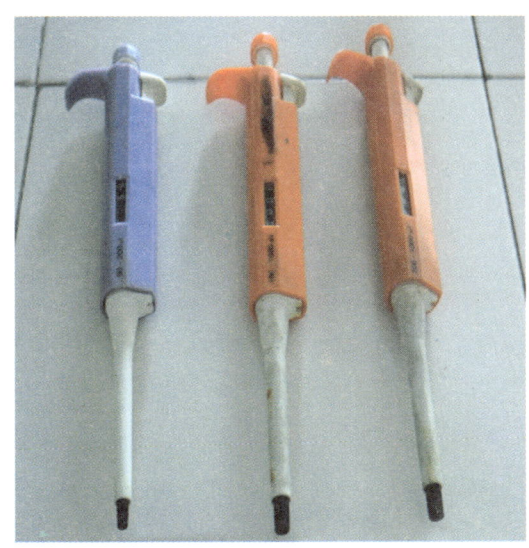

Autopipettes

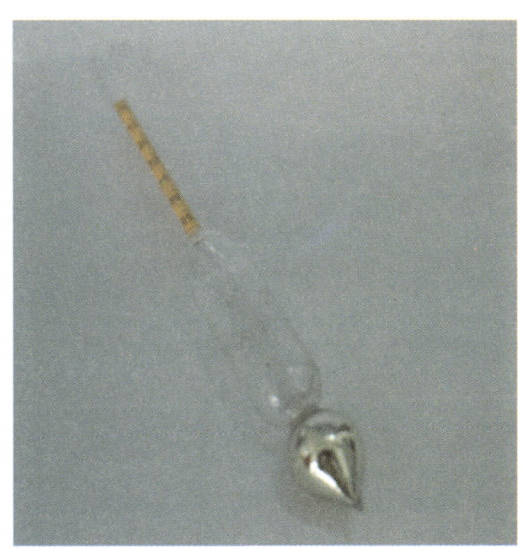

Urinometer

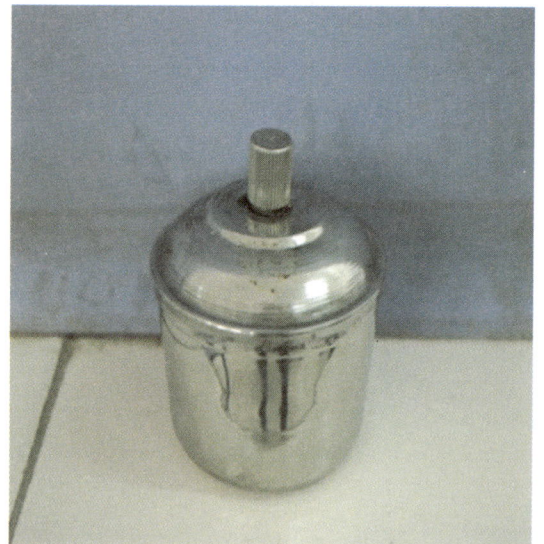

Bunsen burner

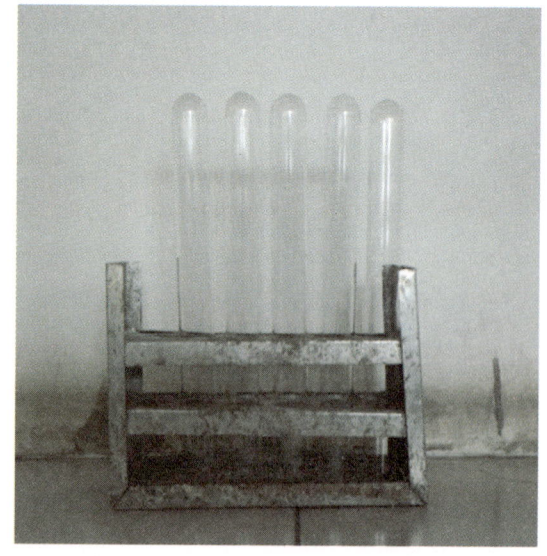

Test tubes with rack

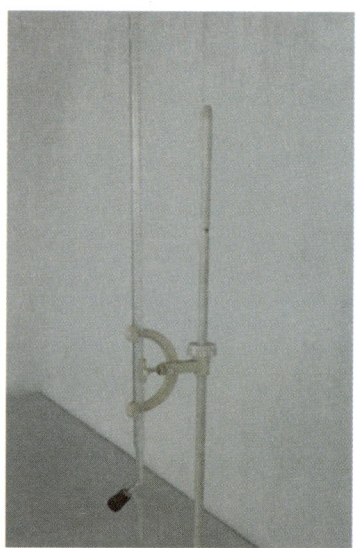

Burette

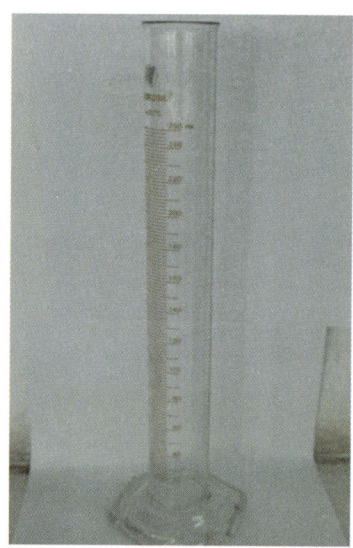

Measuring cylinder

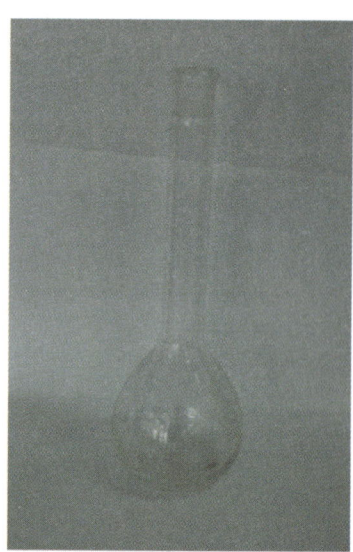

Round bottom flask

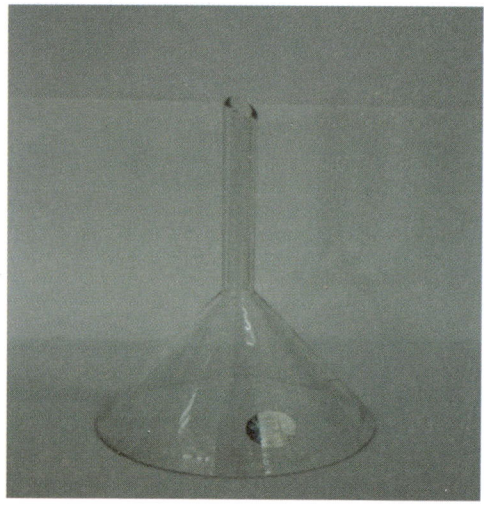

Glass funnel

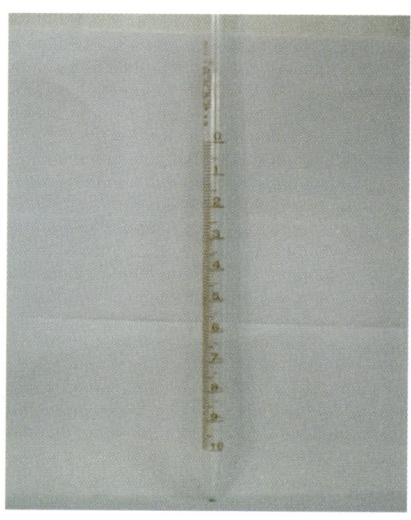

Glass pipette

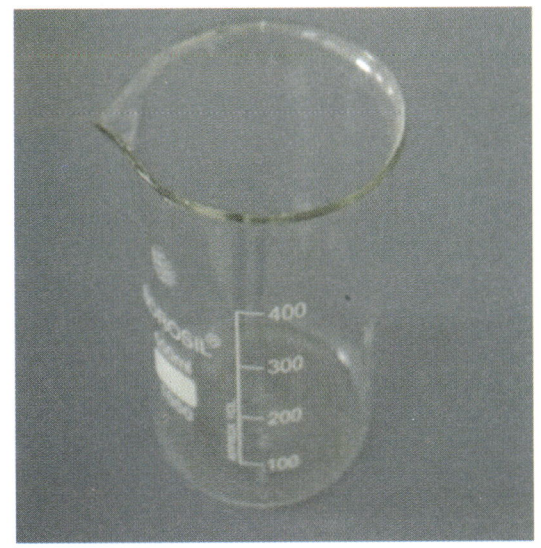

Beaker

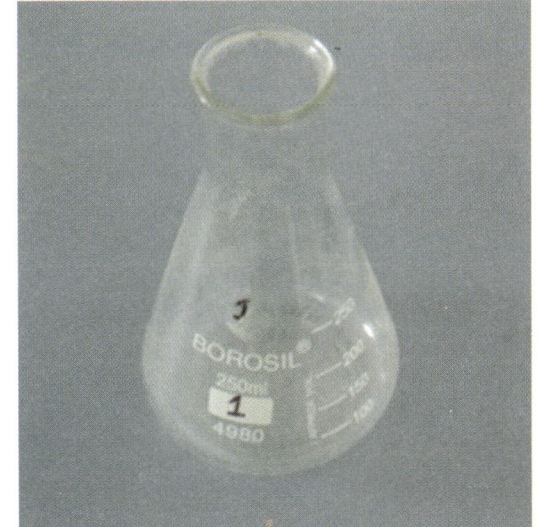

Conical Flask

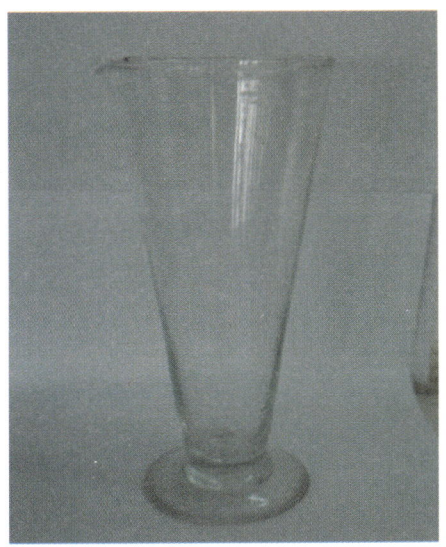

Urine flask

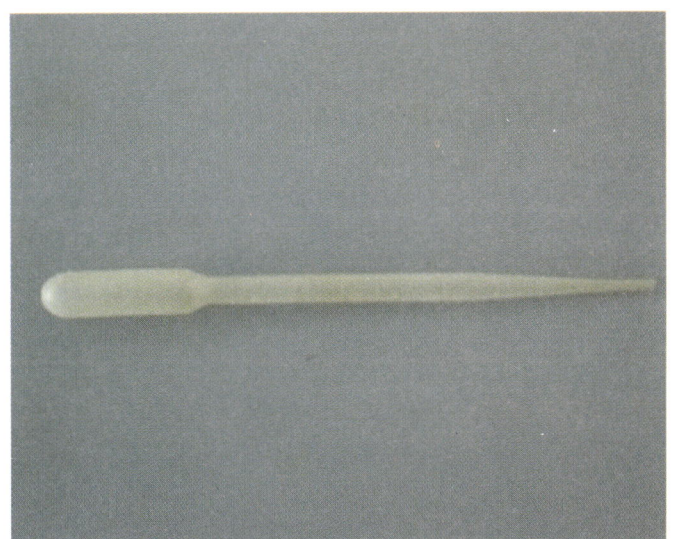

Dropper

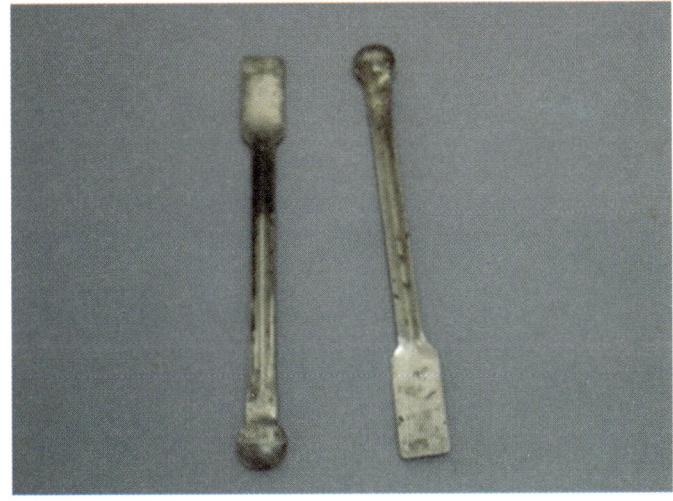

Spatula

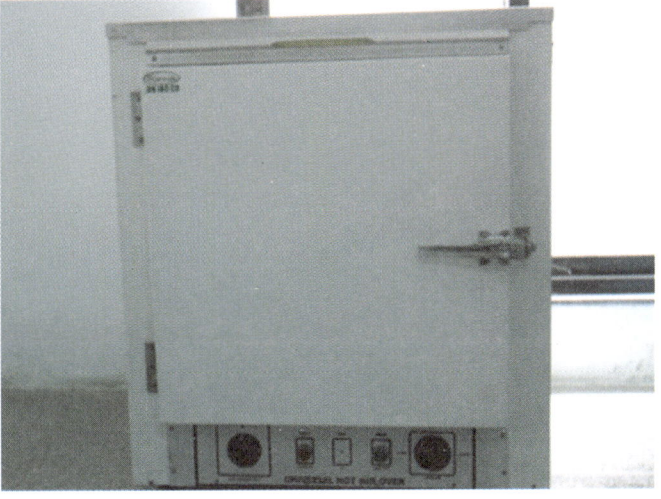

Hot air oven

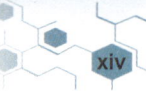

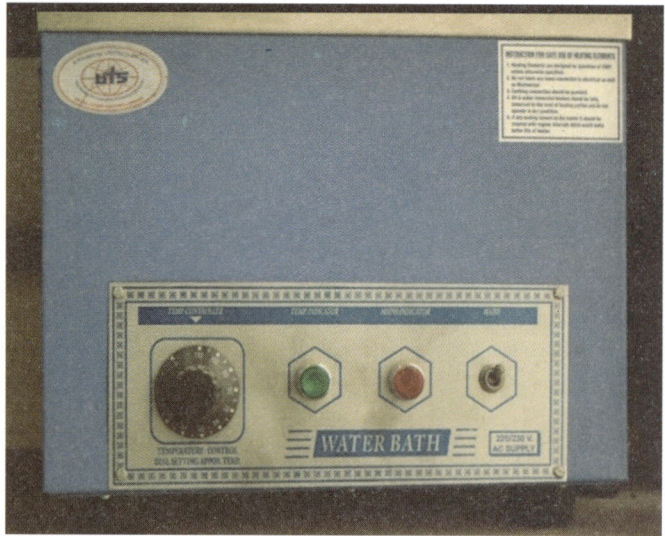

Water bath

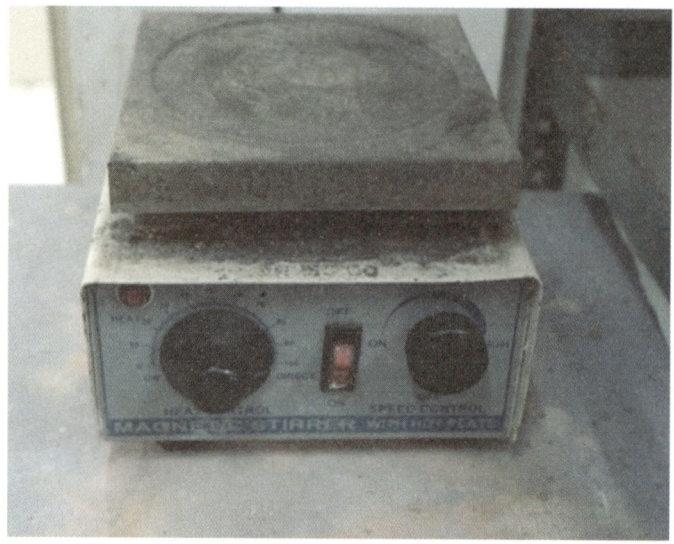

Magnetic stirrer with hot plate

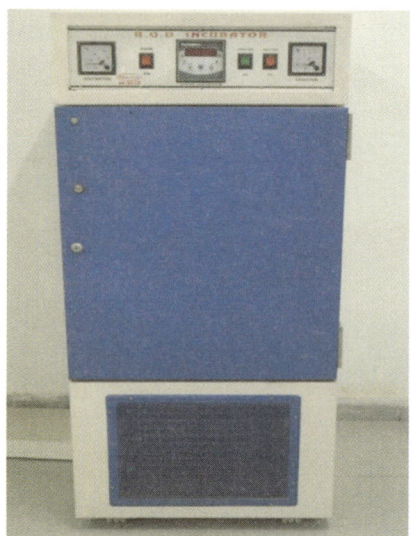

Incubator

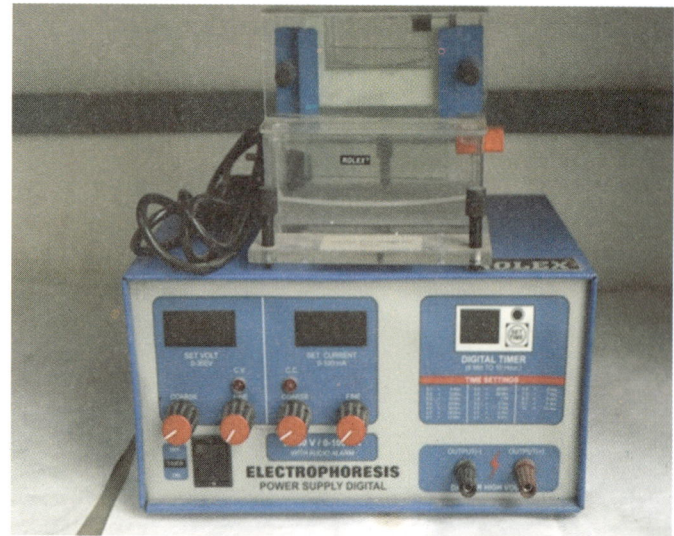

Electrophoresis chamber and power supply

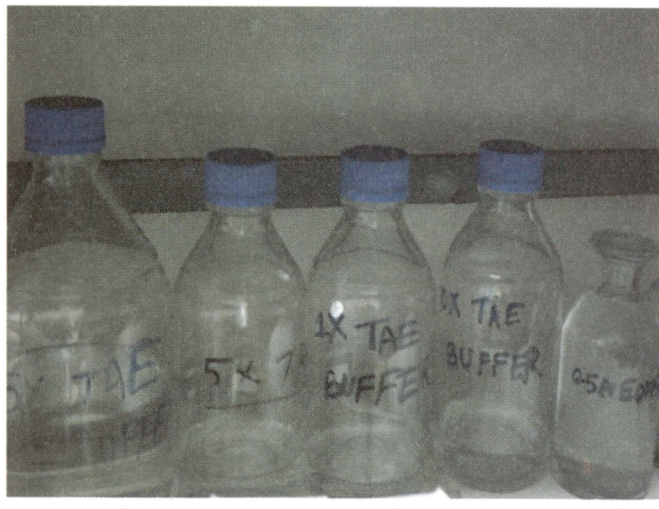

Electrophoresis buffer

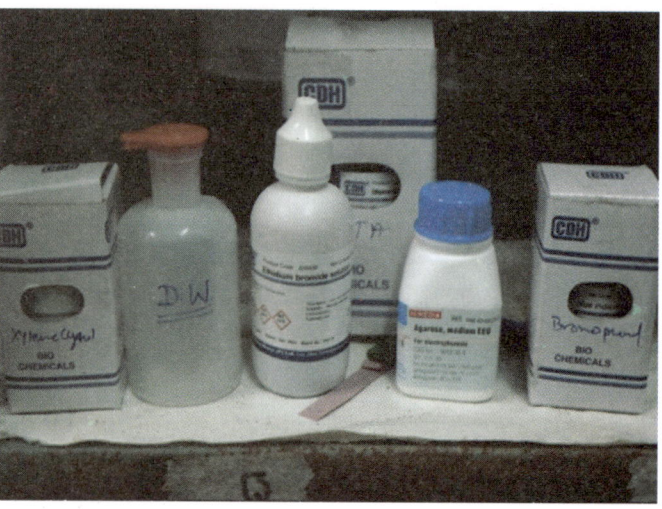

Electrophoresis reagents

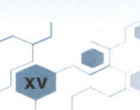

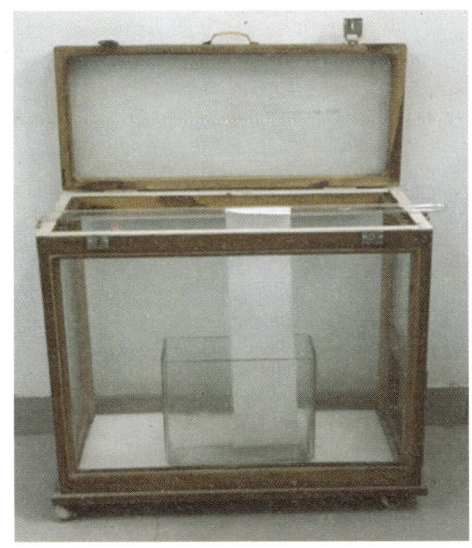

Paper chromatography

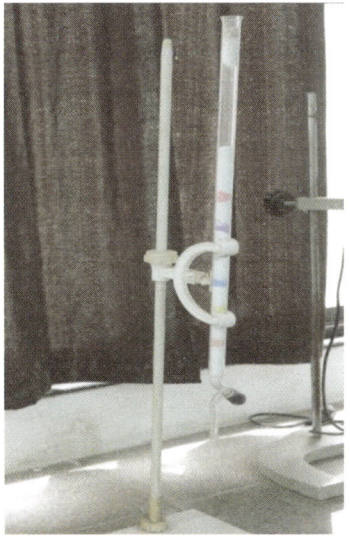

Column chromatography

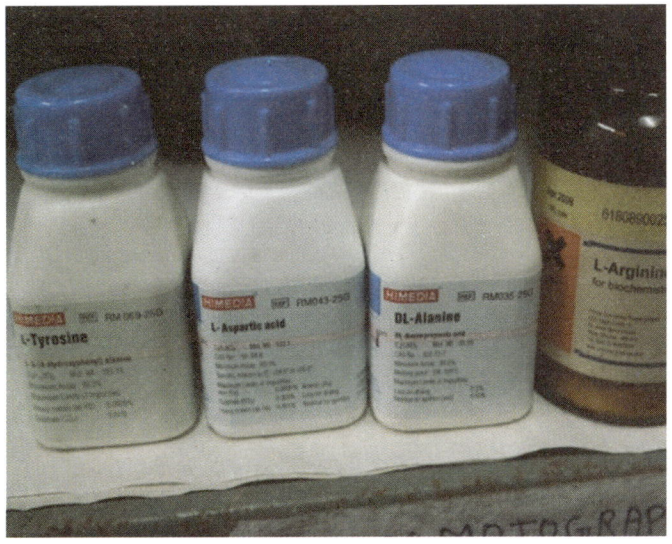

Amino acids used in chromatography

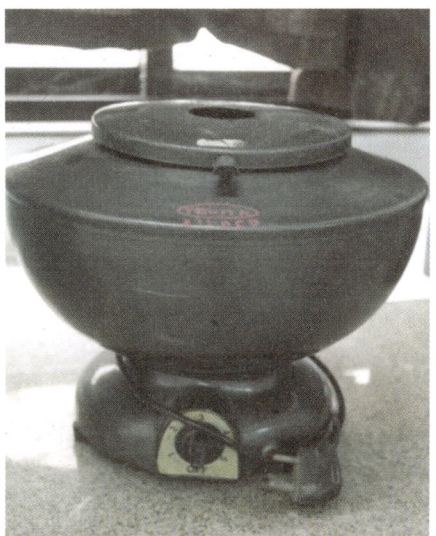

Centrifuge machine

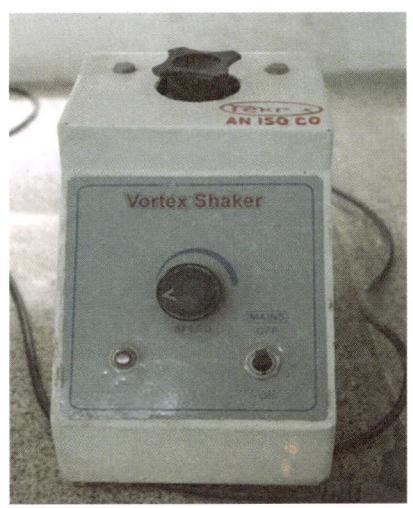

Vortex mixture

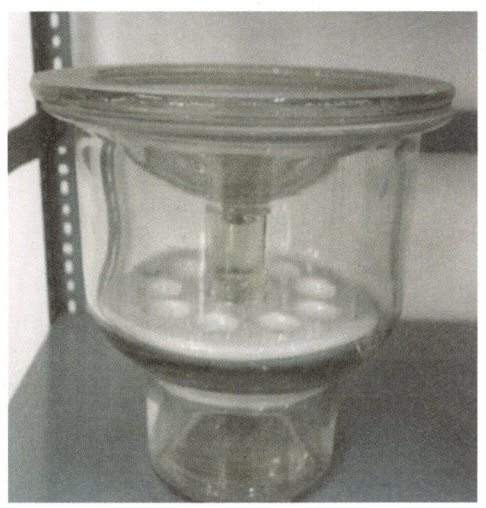

Desicator

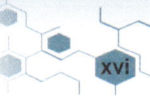

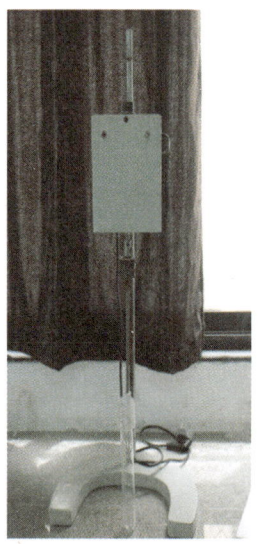

Tissue homogenizer

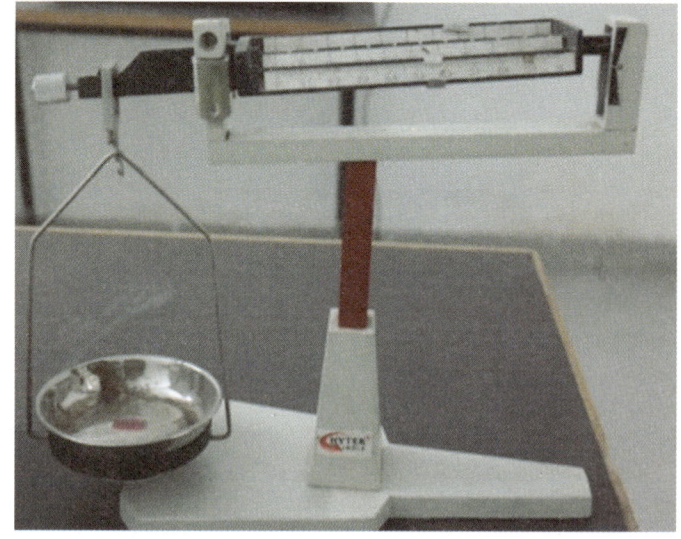

Single pan balance

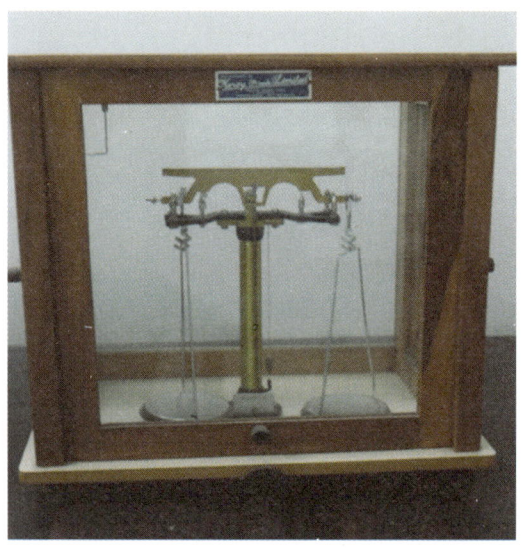

Balance

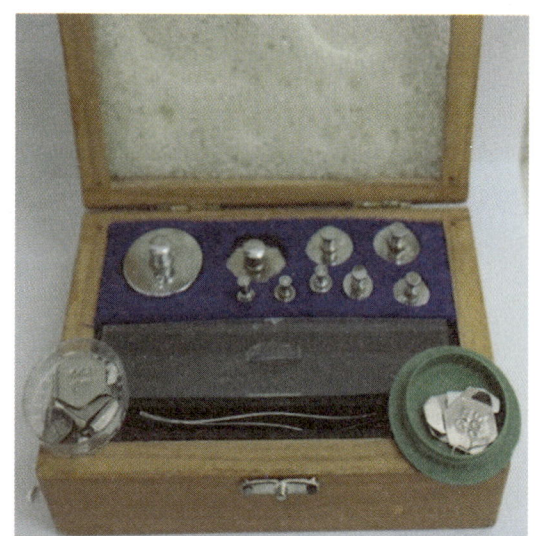

Weights

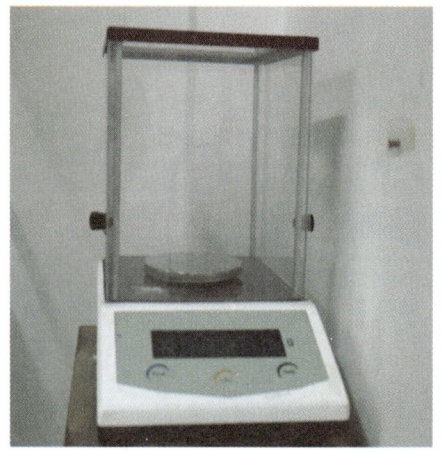

Digital balance

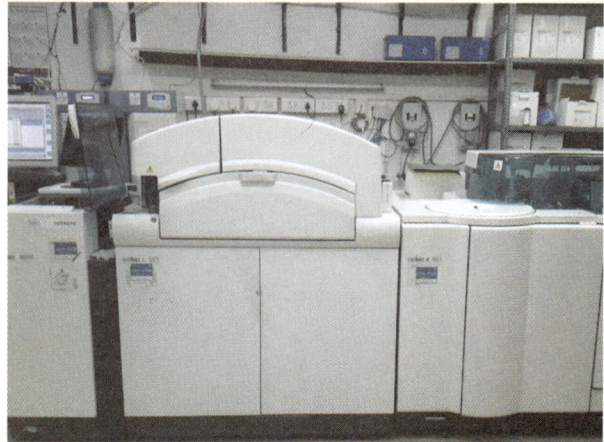

Auto analyzer

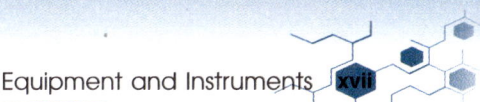

Write Down the Uses and Principle of Each of the Instruments

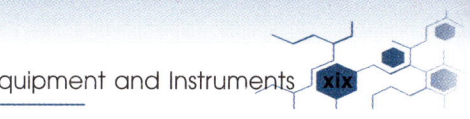

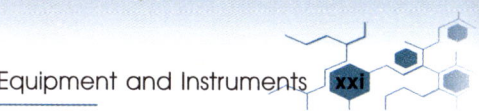

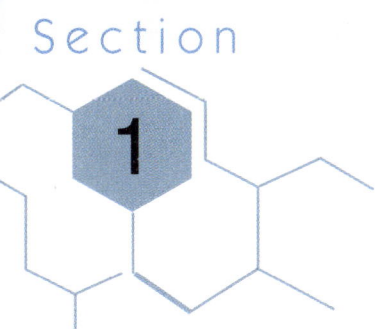
Qualitative Analysis

1. Carbohydrate Analysis
2. Lipids Analysis
3. Protein Analysis
4. Urine Analysis

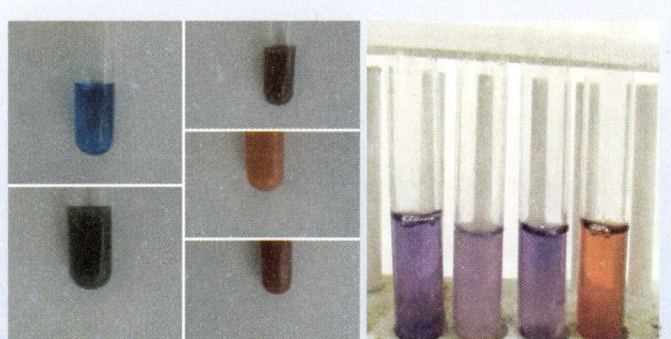

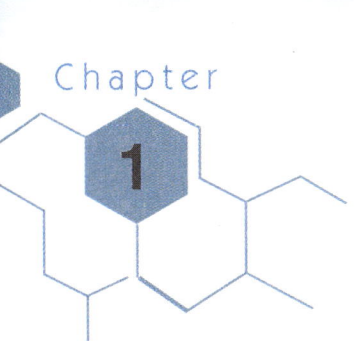

Carbohydrate Analysis

Definition

- Carbohydrates are aldehyde or ketone derivatives of polyhydroxy alcohols.
- Their main function is to provide energy.
- Glucose is the main form of carbohydrate absorb from the gut.
- Humans can synthesize glucose from non-carbohydrate sources like lactate, glucogenic amino acids, propionic acid, glycerol, pyruvate by a process known as gluconeogenesis.

Oligosaccharides: Made up of less than ten monosaccharide subunits.

Classification of Carbohydrates

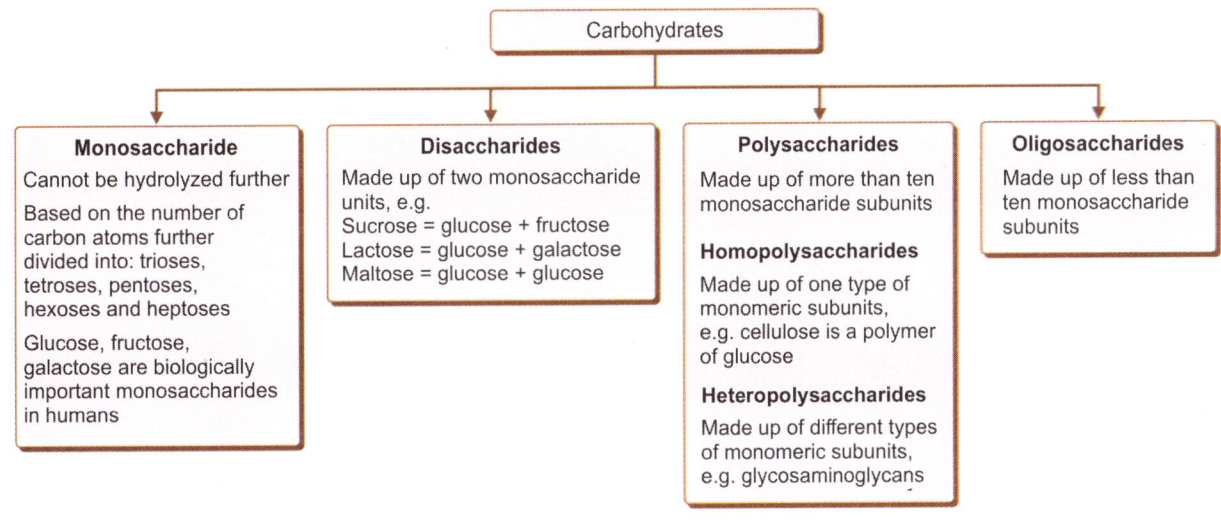

Identification of unknown carbohydrates

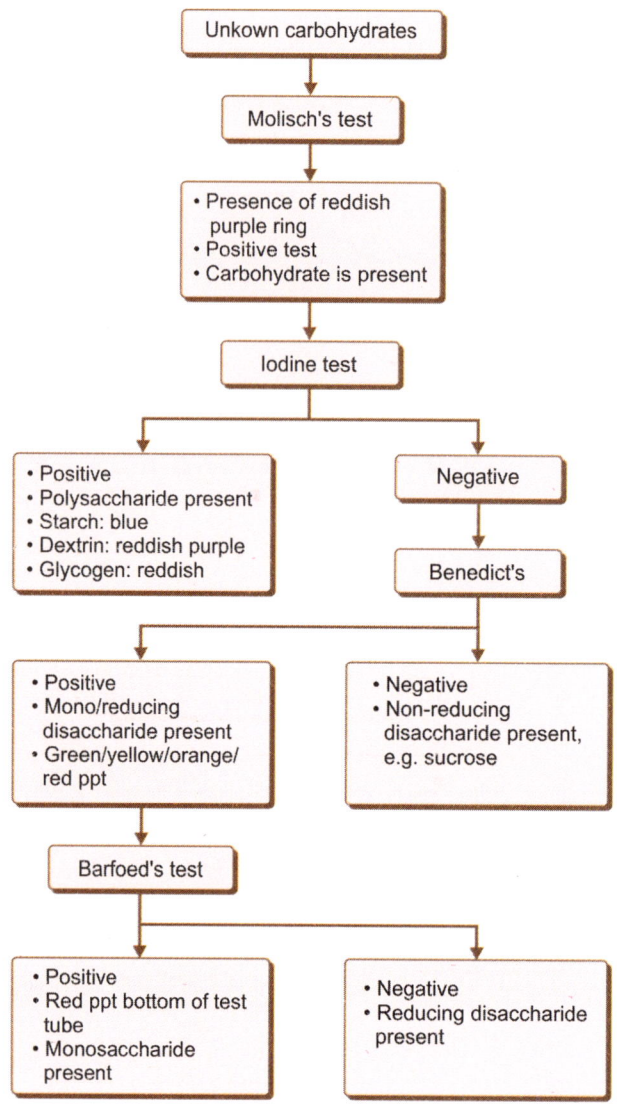

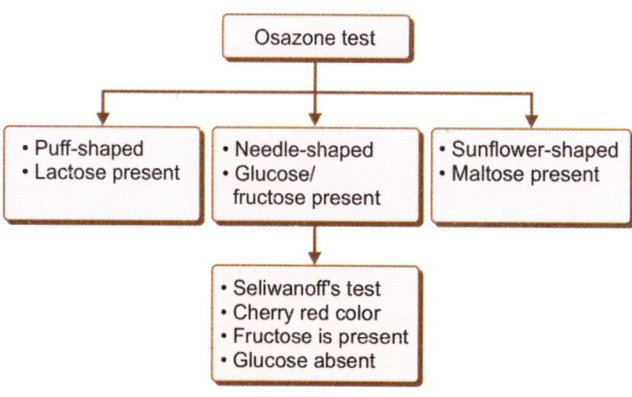

Experiment	Principle	Observation		Inference
Molisch's test (α-naphthol reaction)				
3 ml sugar solution + Molisch reagent (α-naphthol) + Conc sulfuric acid	Conc acid dehydrates sugar to form furfural/furfural derivatives which form complex with molisch reagent	Violet/purple ring at the junction of two liquids (Fig. 1.2)		Carbohydrates present in given solution
Iodine test				
3 ml polysaccharide solution + 0.05N iodine soln 2 drops	Formation of adsorption complex between polysaccharide and iodine	Starch Glycogen Dextrin (Fig. 1.3)	*Colour* Blue Reddish Reddish brown	Polysaccharide is present
Benedict's test				
5 ml benedict reagent + 8 drops sugar soln + Boil for 2 min Benedict reagent: copper sulfate, sodium citrate, sodium carbonate	Reducing sugars have free aldehyde or ketone group, which reduces metallic ions. Benedict reagent has cupric ion which is reduced to cuprous ion	*Colour* Green Yellow Orange Red ppt (Fig. 1.4)	*Conn sugar* 0.5 g >0.5–1 g >1–2 g > 2g	Reducing sugars present
Barfoed test				
5 ml barfoed reagent + 0.5 ml sugar soln + Put in boiling water bath for 2 min	In acid medium free aldehyde or keto group reduces cupric ion into cuprous ion	Red ppt at the bottom of the test tube (Fig. 1.5)		Monosaccharides are present
Osazone test				
5 ml sugar solution + 300 mg phenyl hydrazine mixture + Heat in boiling water bath (15–45 min depends on type of sugar) Cool at room temperature Avoid rapid cooling	Carbonyl carbon and adjacent cabon react with phenyl hydrazine to form phenyl hydrazone, phenyl hydrazone reacts with two molecules of phenyl hydrazine to form osazones	Lactose Puff-shaped Maltose Sunflower-shaped Glucose Needle-shaped Fructose Needle-shaped (Fig. 1.7–1.9)		Confirms the presence of lactose, maltose, glucose and fructose
Seliwanoff's test				
3 ml Seliwanoff's reagent + 5 drops fructose + Heat to just boil	Seliwanoff reagent is resorcinol in dil HCl keto group are readily dehydrated by dil HCl to from hydroxymethylfurfural, which condenses with resorcinol to form red complex	Cherry red color (Fig. 1.6)		Fructose is present
Inversion test				
5 ml sucrose soln + 2 drops conc HCl + Boil for 2 mins and divide into two parts Part 1: Perform Benedict's test Part 2: Perform Seliwanoff's test	Sucrose hydrolyze into glucose and fructose when boiled with conc HCl	Part 1: Positive Benedict test Part 2: Positive Seliwanoff's test	Sucrose is present	

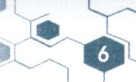

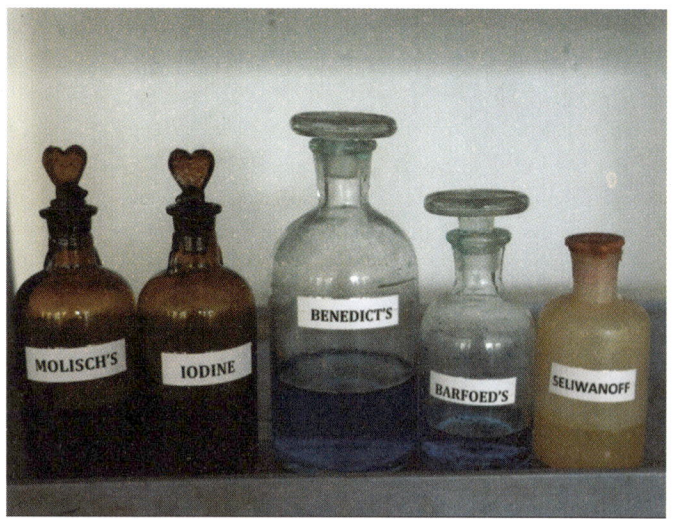

Fig. 1.1: Reagents for carbohydrates identification

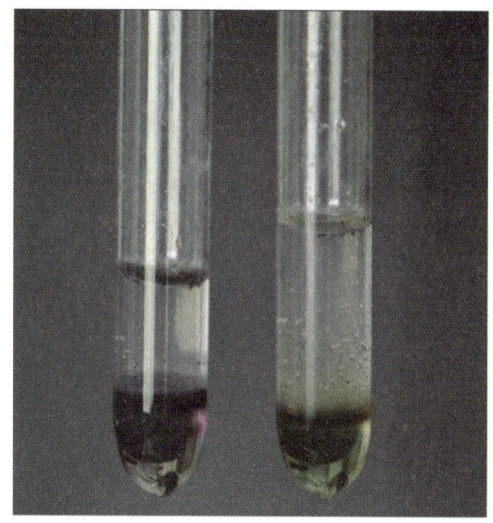

Fig. 1.2: Molisch's test

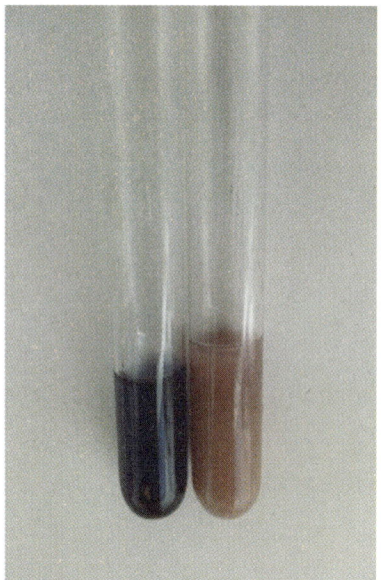

Fig. 1.3: Iodine test

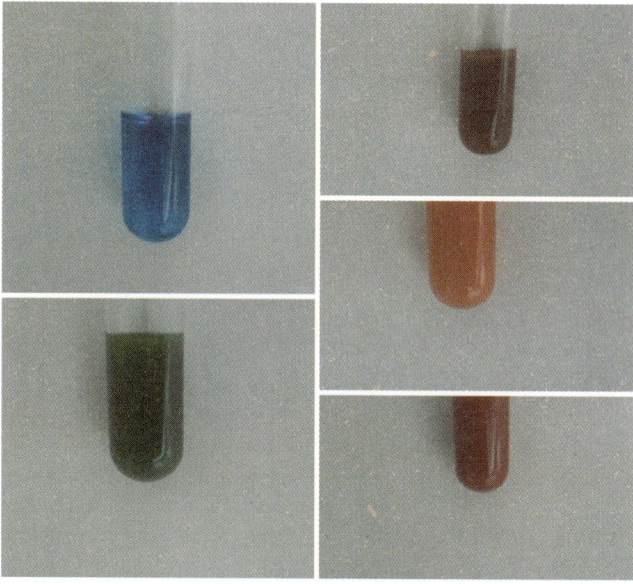

Fig. 1.4: Benedict test: Green, yellow, orange, red

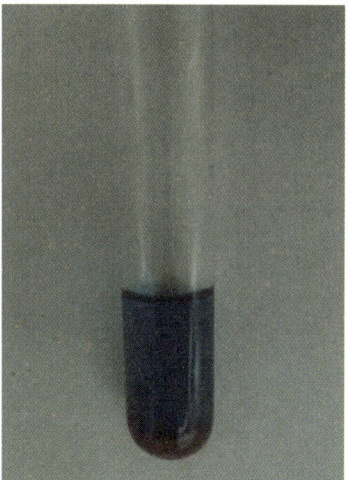

Fig. 1.5: Barfoed's test

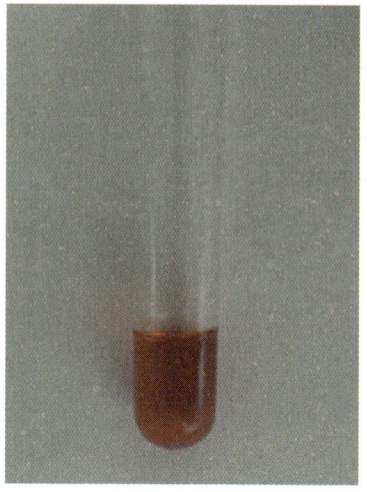

Fig. 1.6: Seliwanoff's test

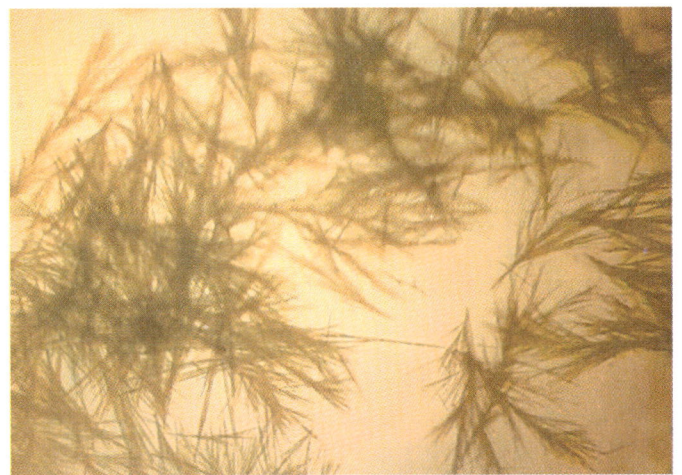

Fig. 1.7: Glucose, fructose-osazone

Fig. 1.8: Maltose- osazone

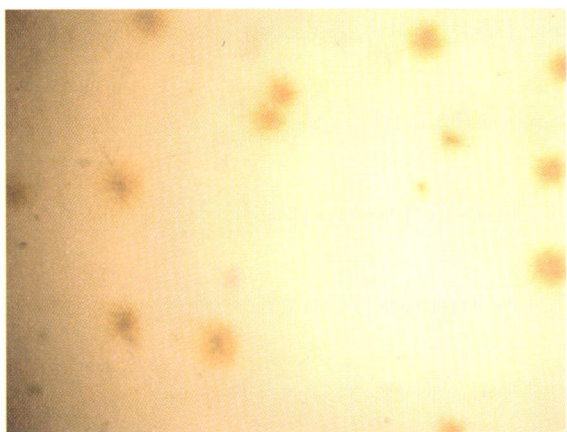

Fig. 1.9: Lactose-osazone

VIVA VOCE

Q1. Name of the group test of carbohydrates.

Ans. Molisch's test

Q2 Why Benedict test is semiquantative test?

Ans. Color of precipitate indicate quantity of sugar in solution.

Q3. Name of test for polysaccharides.

Ans. Iodine Test.

Q4. How to differentiate monosaccharide's glucose and fructose?

Ans. By Seliwanoff's test is positive for fructose.

Q5. Different shape of crystal by osazone test.

Ans. Needle shape—Glucose, fructose
Sunflower shape—Maltose
Cotton ball shape—Lactose

Q.6. Name of common sugar.

Ans. Sucrose

Q7. Carbohydrates preferred in diabetic patients.

Ans. Polysaccharides.

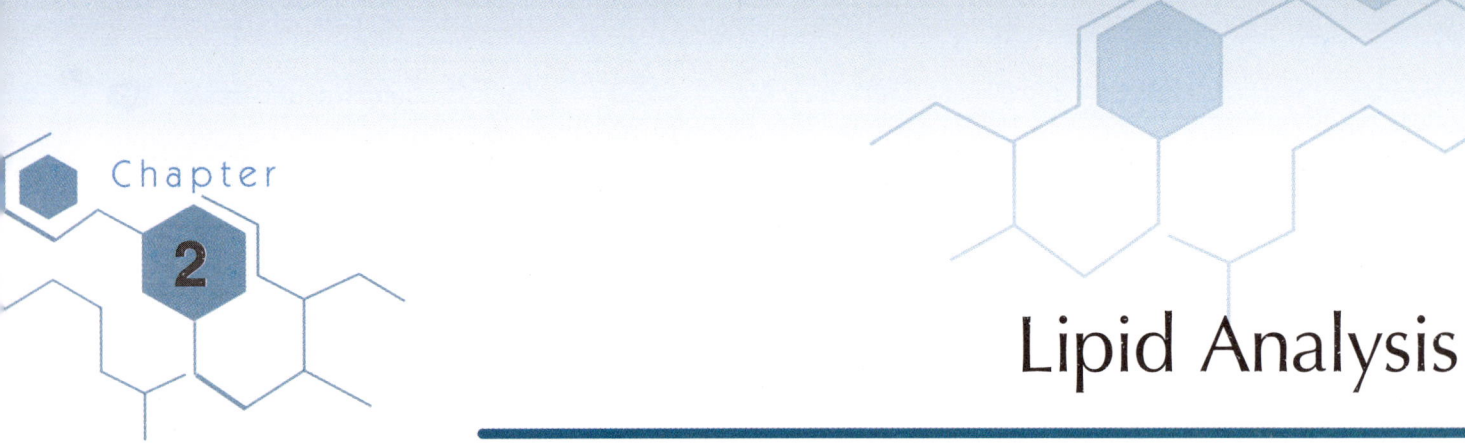

Lipid Analysis

Definition: Lipids are esters of fatty acids with alcohol, which are soluble in organic solvents and insoluble in water.

Classification of Lipids

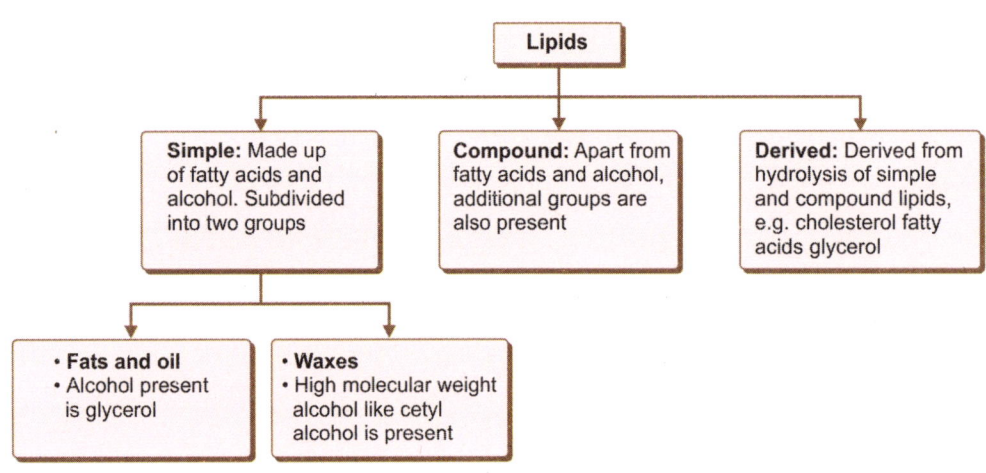

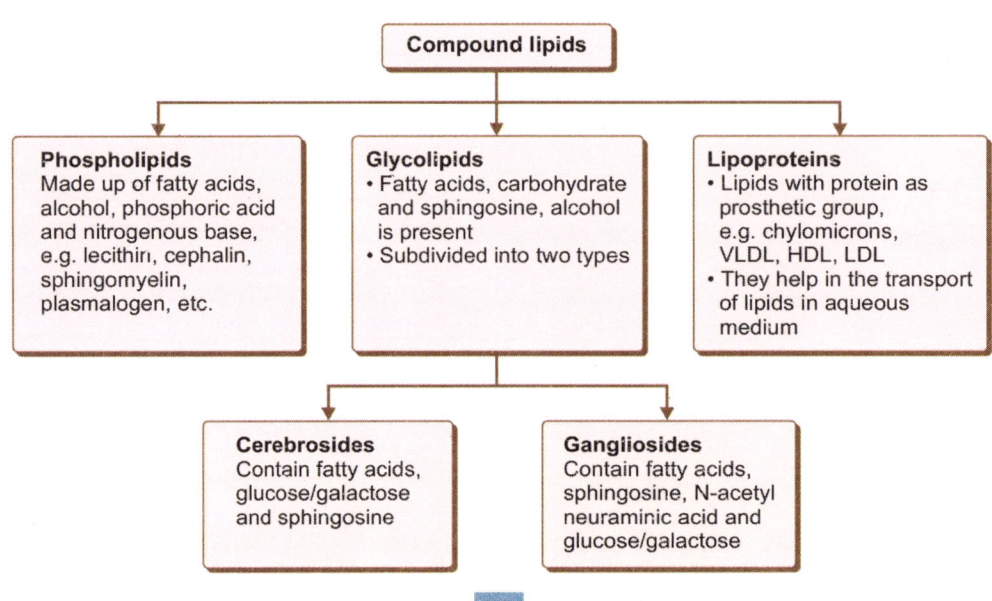

Test	Principle	Observation	Inference
Solubility test: Reagents (ether, chloroform, benzene, CCl₄) **Procedure:** Take 4 test tube and fill 3 ml of water, ether chloroform, benzene CCl₄ in each test tube respectively + Add 5 drops of oil into each test tube + Shake well and allow to stand	This test is based on solubility of lipid in organic solvents and insoluble in water	Oil and water separate quickly in 1st test tube whereas clear solutions are formed in the case of organic solvents	Lipids are insoluble in water and soluble in organic solvents
Saponification test: **Procedure:** Take 5 drop oil and 5 ml of alkali in test tube. Keep test tube in boiling water bath and boil it till the solution become soapy + Cool it take out test tube and add CaCl₂	When oil and fat are boiled with alkali than both are hydrolyzed and liberated fatty acid form salts with alkali called soap and process is known as saponification	A white ppt of insoluble calcium soap is formed	Calcium salt of fatty acid is formed
Emulsification test: **Reagents** (0.5% Na₂CO₃ solution in water + 5% of Bile salt solution) **Procedure:** Take 5 ml of each water bile salt, Na₂CO₃ soap solution in separate + Add 5 drop of oil each + In first tube oil and water layer separates immediately indicating. Emulsion is unstable but in case of Na₂CO₃ layer separate longer time indicating emulsion is more stable	When oil and water are shaken together the oil is broken down into small droplets which are dispersed in water. This is known as oil in water emulsion. The water due to their high surface tension has a tendency to close together and separate as a layer. Bile salt, Na₂CO₃, soap solution lowers the surface tension so they are best emulsifying agents	• Oil and water separate quickly • Separation does not take place with soap, bile salt, Na₂CO₃	• Emulsification is unstable • Emulsification is stable with soap, bile salt, Na₂CO₃
Grease spot test reagent: (Ether) **procedure:** Take 3 ml of ether in test tube + Add 5 drop of oil to it shake well and put 1–2 drop of solution on filter paper wait 5	All lipids are grease in nature so this test is used as a group test for lipid	Ether evaporates and leaving behind a translucent spot on paper (Fig. 2.3)	Grease nature of lipid

Glycerol Analysis

Test	Principle	Observation	Inference
Dunstan's test Reagents: (borax solution + phenolphthalein indicator) **Procedure:** 3 ml of borax solution in test tube + add drop of phenolphthalein indicator pink color produced indicate medium is alkaline + add 20% glycerol drop by drop until pink color disappears indicate medium is acidic. Heat again until pink color reappears that indicate medium has become alkaline again	Borax hydrolyzed into NaOH (strong base) and boric acid (weak acid) after addition of glycerol it react with boric acid and forms strong acid (glyceroboric acid)	Medium is alkaline-pink color disappear. Medium is acidic than color will reappear (Fig. 2.1)	Presence of glycerol
Acrolein test: Reagents- solid $KHSO_4$ **Procedure:** Take dry test + add 1–2 drop of glycerol + add pinch of $KHSO_4^+$ heat it	On heating with $KHSO_4$ glycerol is dehydrated to form an unsaturated aldehyde (acrolein)	Pungent smell is produced	Presence of glycerol

Cholesterol Analysis

Procedure	Principle	Observation	Inference
Salkowski's test Reagent: con H_2SO_4 **Procedure:** Take 2 ml of cholesterol in dry test tube + add 2 ml of conc H_2SO_4 shake well and allow to stand	When sample is dissolved in chloroform and equal volume of H_2SO_4 is added. If cholesterol is present solution become blue red and change to violet red and H_2SO_4 become red with green fluorescence	Two layer separated chloroform layer-cherry red (Fig. 2.2) acid layer–green fluorescence	Presence of cholesterol
Libermann-Burchard's test reagent: Con H_2SO_4 Acetic anhydride **Procedure:** Take 3 ml of cholesterol in dry test tube + add 10 drop of acetic anhydride + add 1–2 drops of con H_2SO_4 mix well	Cholesterol is dehydrated by con H_2SO_4 and acetic anhydride leading to formation of 2,4 or 3,5 cholestadienes	Red color develops followed by blue and finally whole solution becomes green	Presence of cholesterol

Test for Unsaturation (Hubl's Iodine Test)

Procedure	Principle	Observation	Inference
Hubl's iodine test) Reagents-iodine 26 gm Mercuric chloride 30 gm C_2H_5OH 1000 ml. Procedure 3 ml of $CHCl_3$ + add Hubl's reagent drop by drop	Unsaturated fatty acid absorb iodine at double bonds until all the bonds are saturated with iodine	Color of iodine disappears	Show degree of unsaturation

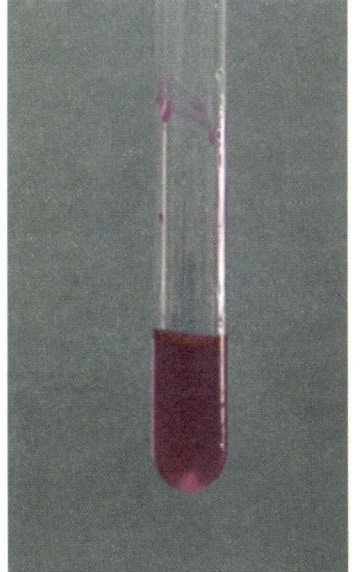
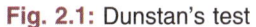

Fig. 2.1: Dunstan's test

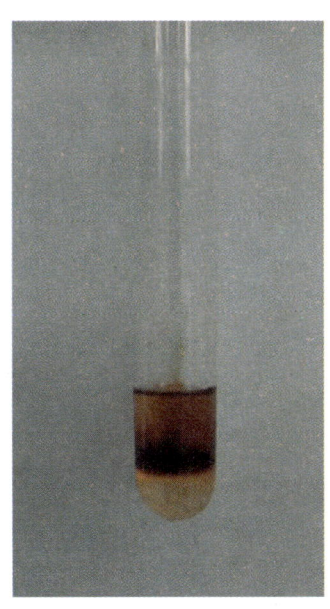

Fig. 2.2: Salkowski's test

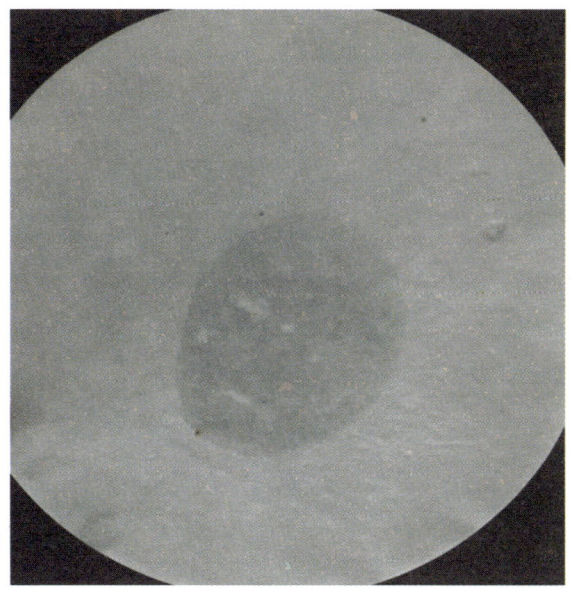

Fig. 2.3: Grease spot test

VIVA VOCE

Q1. Name of essential fatty acids.

Ans. Lionlic acid, linoleic acid.

Q2. Name of the test for cholesterol.

Ans. Salkowski, Liberman-Burchard reaction.

Q3. Name of ring present in cholesterol.

Ans. CPPP (cyclopentaperhydrophenenthrene).

Q4. Name of the test for unsaturation of fatty acids.

Ans. Hubl's iodine test.

Q5. What is the importance of emulsification?

Ans. Digestion of lipids.

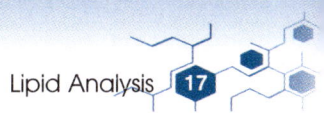

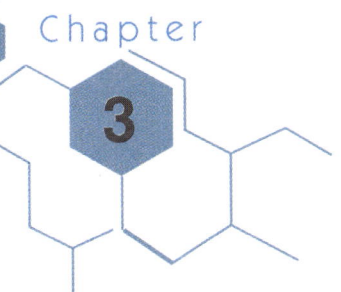

Protein Analysis

Definition: Polymers of L-amino acids linked by peptide bond.

Classification of Proteins

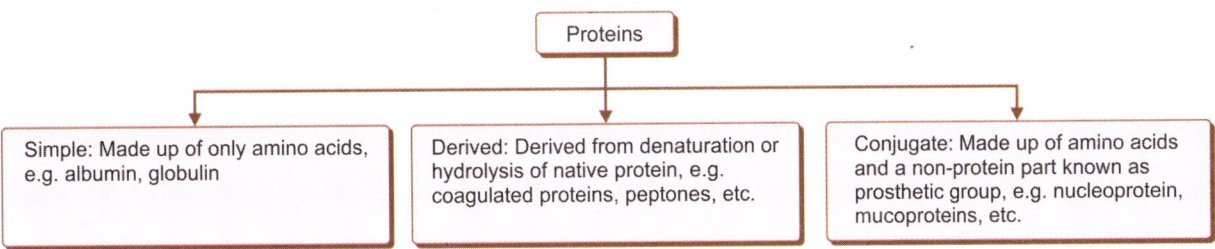

Color Reactions

A. Biuret Test, Ninhydrin Test (Group Color Reaction for Amino Acids)

Test procedure	Principle	Observation	Inference
Biuret test **Reagents: 40%** NaOH **Procedure:** 2 ml protein solution + 1 ml NaOH mix + 1–2 drops of 0.5% $CuSO_4$	Violet color formation because of peptide linkage of protein with $CuSO_4$ in alkali medium provided by NaOH	Violet color presence (Fig. 3.1)	Peptide linkage, presence of protein
Ninhydrin **Reagents:** 0.1% Freshly prepared ninhydrin solution **Procedure:** 1 ml protein solution + 1 ml freshly prepared 0.1% ninhydrin solution mix and boil for 1 min, cool	Heating with ninhydrin (oxidizing agent) α amino acids give purple color	Violet—purple color (Fig. 3.2)	Presence of α amino acids **Exception:** Proline and hydroxyl proline

B. Xanthoproteic, Millon Nasse's, Hopkin's Cole's (Aromatic Amino Acids)

Test procedure	Principle	Observation	Inference
Xanthoproteic Reagents: Con. HNO_3, 40% NaOH **Procedure:** 3 ml protein solution + 1 ml HNO_3 heat for 1 min yellow, cool + 2 ml 40% NaOH mix-orange color	Heating of aromatic amino acids with HNO_3 lead to nitration of benzene group of amino acids, by ionization it give orange color	Yellow to dark yellow convert in to orange color (Fig. 3.3)	Presence of aromatic amino acids

Contd...

Test procedure	Principle	Observation	Inference
Millon Nasse's (tyrosine) reagents: 15% $HgSO_4$ in 6N H_2SO_4 (Millon Nasse's reagent), $NaNO_2$ freshly prepared **Procedure:** 4 ml solution + 1.5 ml Millon's reagent- Boil-cool 1 ml $NaNO_2$	Mercuration and nitration of phenolic group—development of color	Red-pink color developed in precipitate and solution (Fig. 3.4)	Tyrosine presence
Hopkin cole (aldehyde) reagents: Conc H_2SO_4, dilute formaldehyde **Procedure:** 2 ml protein solution + 1 ml formaldehyde mix + 2 ml H_2SO_4 along the side wall of test tube slowly	Indole ring combine with formaldehyde in presence of con H_2SO_4—violet ring	Violet ring at the junction (Fig. 3.5)	Tryptophan presence

C. Sakaguchi's (Test for Arginine)

Test procedure	Principle	Observation	Inference
Sakaguchi reagents: 10% NaOH, α napthol, 10% sodium hypobromite **Procedure:** 3 ml protein solution + 1 ml 10% NaOH mix + 2–3 drop of sodium hypobromite and mix well	Guanido group react with α napthol and sodium hypobromite and give red color complex	Presence of red color (Fig. 3.6)	Guanido group (arginine presence)

D. Lead Sulphide (Test for Sulfur Group)

Test procedure	Principle	Observation	Inference
Lead sulfide (cysteine and cystine) **Reagents:** 40% NaOH, 2% acetate **Procedure:** 3 ml protein + 2.5 ml 40% NaOH boil – 2 min – cool + 3–4 drop lead acetate	In alkali medium sulfur release as sodium sulfide and react with lead acetate form lead sulfide (black-brown color)	Brown black ppt form (Fig. 3.7)	Presence of sulfur con. amino acids (negative for casein and gelatin) lead

E. Neumann's (Test for phosphate group)

Test procedure	Principle	Observation	Inference
Neumann's (casein) Reagents: Ammonium molybdate, methyl red indicator, conc nitric acid, conc ammonia, conc H_2SO_4 **Procedure:** Dry pinch of casein + 6–8 drop of conc H_2SO_4 + 2–3 drop of conc HNO_3^- heat untill colorless. cool + methy indicator with 3 ml water red + ammonia-untill change in yellow + add conc HNO_3^- red, boil for 2 min, 2 ml ammonium molybdate, heat	Heating with conc H_2SO_4 + HNO_3 casein digested phosphorus remove, then react with ammonium molybdate its form ammonium phoshph-omolybdate-canary yellow color	Canary yellow color (Fig. 3.8)	Phosphorus group present

F. Coagulation and precipitation reaction

Test procedure	Principle	Observation	Inference
Heat coagulation 2/3 test tube with protein solution incline heat upper part + acetic acid	Denaturation of protein	Dense coagulum formed at upper part not dissolved adding of acetic acid (Fig. 3.9)	Presence of albumin and globulin (protein)
Precipitation reagents: Ammonium sulfate, $AgNO_3$, $HgNO_3$ sulfosalicylic acid	Shell of hydration, electrical charge	White ppt form	Albumin, casein, gelatin
Full saturation procedure: 3 ml protein + solid ammonium sulfate till saturation–allow to standing			
Half saturation procedure: 3 ml protein solution + saturated 3 ml, mix well-standing	Shell of hydration, electrical charge	White ppt form	Casein, gelatin
Heavy metals procedure: 3 ml protein + drop by drop heavy metals salt till ppt formation	Negatively charged protein react with metal and neutralize form ppt	Ppt form	Protein presence
Alkaloid reagents procedure: 3 ml protein + sulfosalicylic acid mixing	Acid base reaction form insoluble salt	White turbidity	Protein presence

G. Identification of Unknown Protein

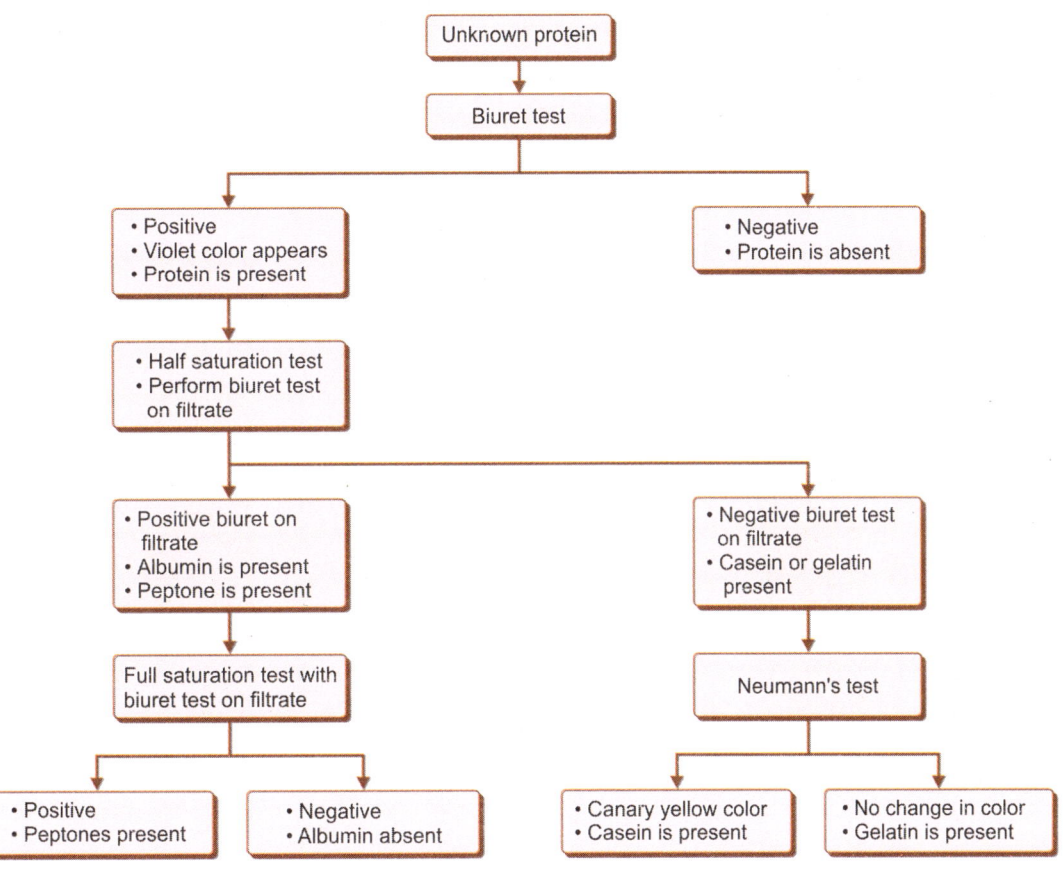

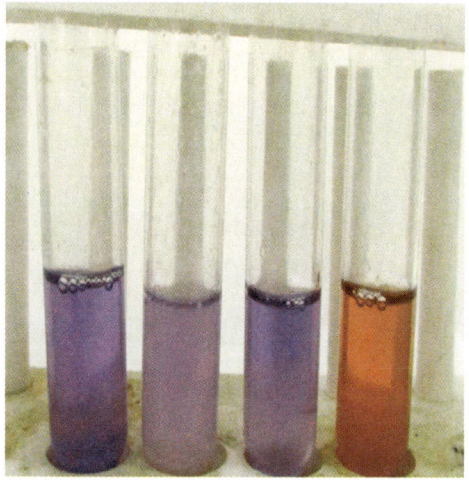

Fig. 3.1: Biuret test:
Albumin, casein, gelatin, peptone

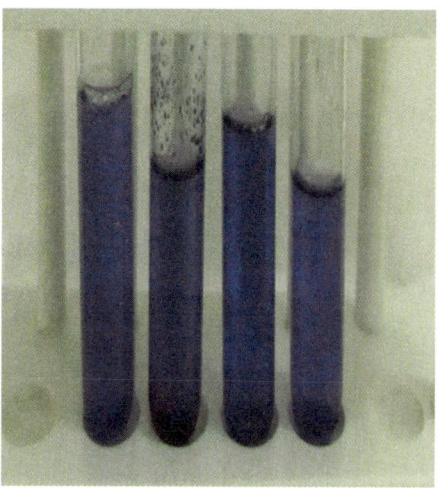

Fig. 3.2: Ninhydrin test:
Albumin, casein, gelatin, peptone

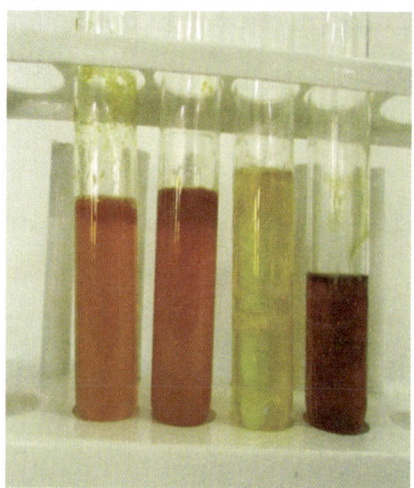

Fig. 3.3: Xanthoproteic test:
Albumin, casein, gelatin, peptone

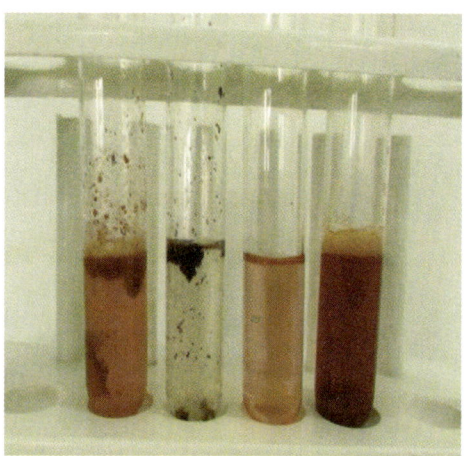

Fig. 3.4: Million Nasse's test:
Albumin, casein, gelatin, peptone

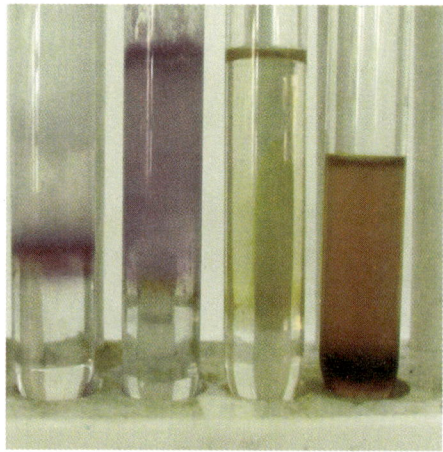

Fig. 3.5: Hopkin's Cole's test:
Albumin, casein, gelatin, peptone

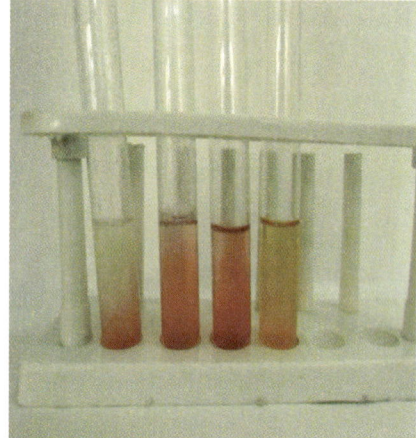

Fig. 3.6: Sakaguchi's test:
Albumin, casein, gelatin, peptone

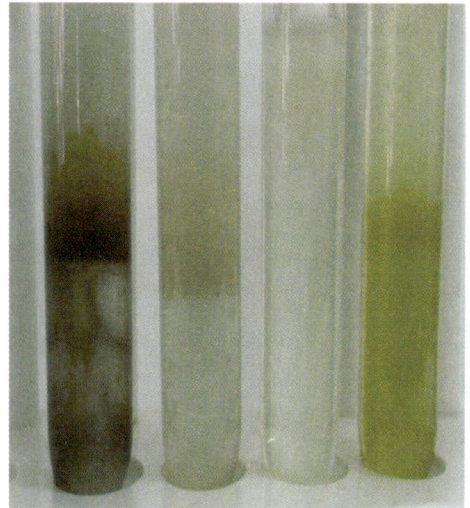

Fig. 3.7: Lead sulphide test:
Albumin, casein, gelatin, peptone

Note: From left to right albumin, casein, gelatin, peptone

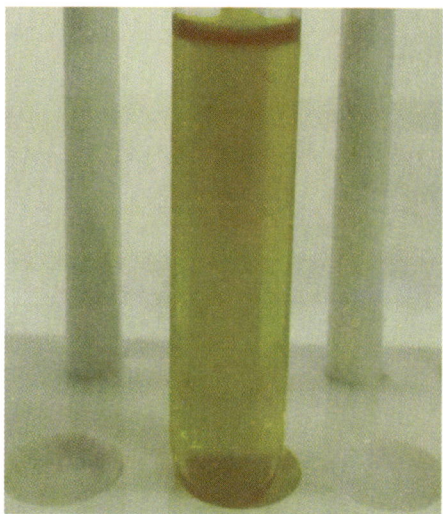

Fig. 3.8: Neumann's test: Casein

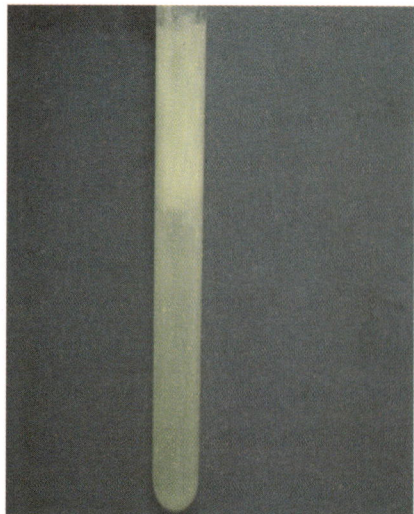

Fig. 3.9: Heat coagulation's test:
Albumin

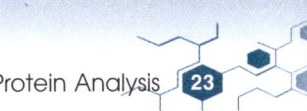

VIVA VOCE

Q1. Name of the group test for proteins.

Ans. Biuret test.

Q2. Name of the test for aromatic ring containing amino acids.

Ans. Xanthoproteic acids.

Q3. Specific test for tyrosine.

Ans. Millons test.

Q4. Test name for tryptophan.

Ans. Hopkin's cole's.

Q5. Specific test for sulphur test.

Ans. Lead acetate.

Q6. Test for casein.

Ans. Neumann's test.

Q7. How to differentiate albumin and gelatin by saturation test?

Ans. Gelatin gives half saturation, while albumin gives full saturation.

Q8. Name of first class protein.

Ans. Albumin.

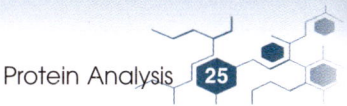

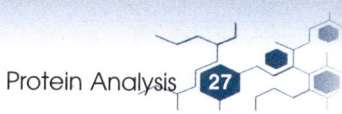

Urine Analysis

NORMAL URINE

Urine is the excretory product of body, formed by kidneys. It is made up of water and water soluble waste products. Examination of urine gives us idea of renal function.

Normal Constituents of Urine

1. Water	90–95%
2. Urea	25–30 gm/day
3. Creatinine	1–1.2 gm/day
4. Uric acid	0.4–0.7 gm/day
5. Sodium	3–3.5 gm/day
6. Potassium	2–2.5 gm/day
7. Chloride	10–15 gm/day
8. Calcium	0.1–0.3 gm/day
9. Phosphate	0.7–1.2 gm/day
10. Sulfate	1–1.2 gm/day
11. Ammonia	0.6–0.8 gm/day

Physical Examination of Normal Urine

1. Appearance	Freshly void urine is clear, it becomes turbid on standing due to precipitation of phosphates
2. Odor	Aromatic odor, which becomes ammonical on standing
3. Color	Straw color
4. Volume	1–2 L/day, depends upon the intake of water
5. pH	Usually acidic, pH ranges from 4.5 to 8 post meal, pH of urine is alkaline; it is called alkaline tide
6. Specific gravity	1.010–1.025, measured with the help of urinometer, it tell us about the concentrating ability of kidneys

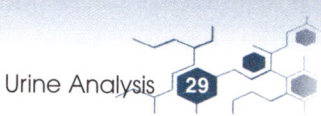

Test	Principle	Observation	Inference
Urea **1. Specific urease test reagents:** Soybean meal, phenol red **Procedure:** 4–5 ml of urine + pinch of soybean meal + 1–2 drop of phenol indicator mix and wait 10 mins	Urease in soybean meal acts on urea and liberate NH_3, which makes the medium alkaline. In alkaline medium phenolphthalein gives red color	Yellow color Red color (Due to NH_3) (Fig. 4.2a)	Presence of urea
2. Sodium hypobromite test reagents: Alkaline hypobromite **Procedure:** 4–5 ml sample + 2 ml alkaline hypobromite + mix	Breakdown of urea and release of nitrogen produce effervescence	Effervescence due to production of nitrogen (Fig. 4.2b)	Presence of urea
Calcium test reagents: Ammonium oxalate **Procedure:** Take 2–3 ml ammonium oxalate + 1–2 ml urine	Formation of calcium oxalate	White ppt of calcium oxalate (Fig. 4.4)	Presence of calcium
Phosphate test reagents: Ammonium molybdate **Procedure:** Take 1–2 ml urine + add con HNO_3 + heat + ammonium molybdate	Formation of phospho-molybdate	Canary yellow ppt (Fig. 4.5)	Presence of phosphate
Creatinine test Jaffe's test reagents: Alkaline picrate **Procedure:** 3–4 ml urine + 1 ml alkaline picrate	Formation of creatinine picrate	Orange red color (Fig. 4.3)	Presence of creatinine
Uric acid Benedict's test reagents: Sodium tungstste, arsenic pentoxide, phosphoric acid, HCl, anhydrous sodium carbonate **Procedure:** 4 ml urine + pinch of sodium carbonate + mix + 4–5 drop of above reagent + mix	In alkaline medium, arsenophosphotungstate of Benedict's uric acid regent is reduced to blue colored arsenophosphotungstate	Blue color develop	Presence of uric acid
Ammonia test reagents: Phenolphthalein indicatior **Procedure:** 9 ml urine + drop of phenolphthalein indicatior + drop of 0.1 N NaOH hold glass rod at the mouth of tube	Ammonia is alkaline in nature which turns phenolphthalein indicator pink	Tip of rod turns pink	Presence of ammonia

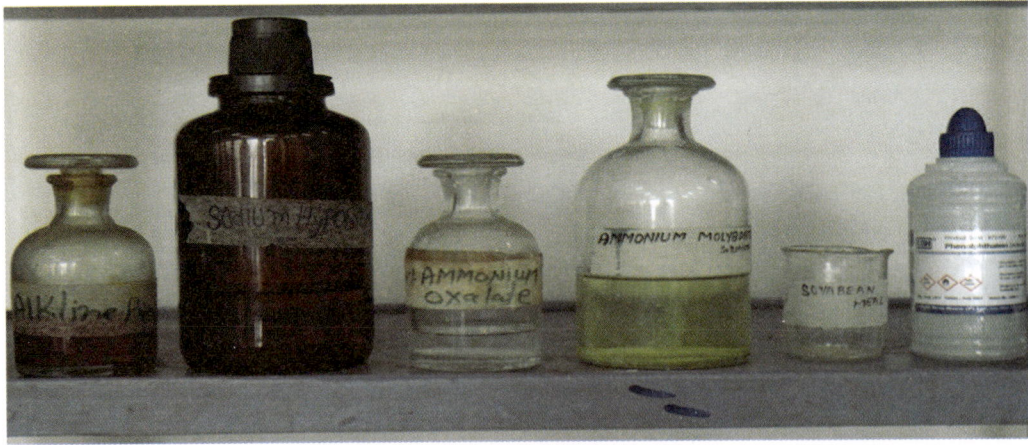

Fig. 4.1: Reagents

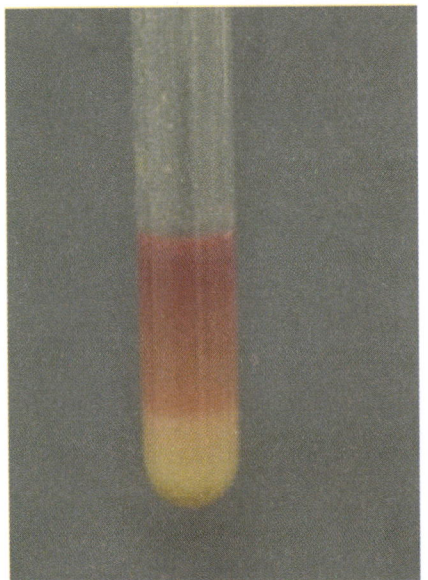

Fig. 4.2a: Test for urea, soybean meal

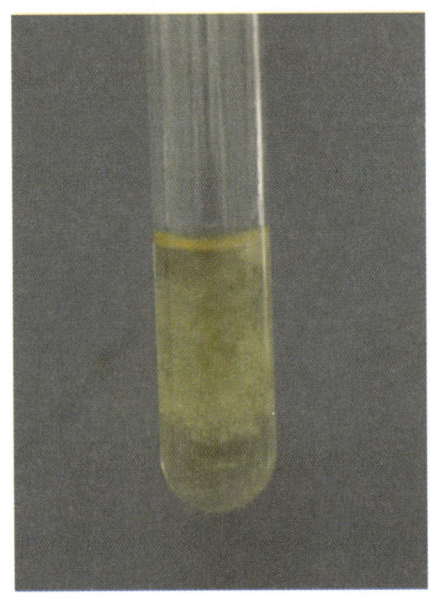

Fig. 4.2b: Sodium hypobromite test

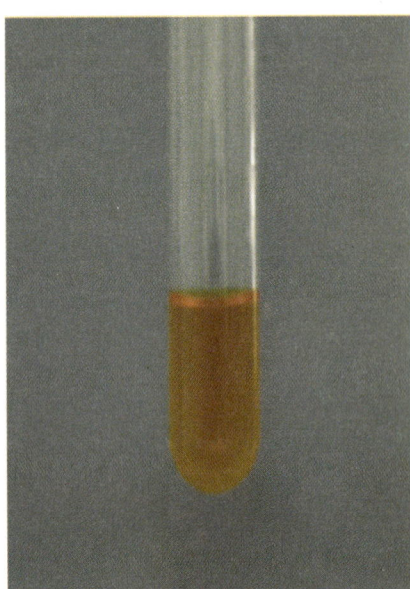

Fig. 4.3: Test for creatinine

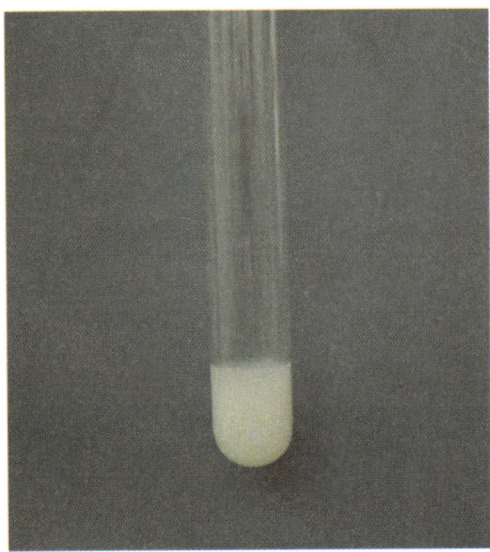

Fig. 4.4: Test for calcium

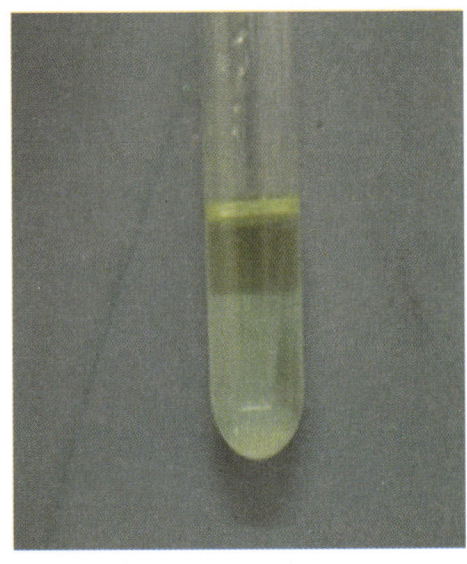

Fig. 4.5: Test for phosphate

PATHOLOGICAL URINE

Physical Examination of Pathological Urine

	Normal	Pathological
Appearance	Clear	a. Turbid in UTI
Odor	Aromatic	a. Fruity in diabetic ketoacidosis, starvation due to presence of ketone bodies
		b. Mousy odor in phenylketonuria
		c. Foul smell in UTI
Color	Straw color	a. Red in hematuria
		b. Brown to black in alkaptonuria
		c. Brown in hemoglobinuria
Volume	1–2 L/day	a. Oliguria <300 ml/day
		b. Polyuria >2500 ml/day seen in diabetes mellitus and diabetes insipidus
		c. Anuria <100 ml/day
pH	4.5–8	a. pH decreases in metabolic acidosis
		b. Increase in pH is seen in metabolic alkalosis and UTI
Specific gravity (SG)	1.010–1.025	a. Isothenuria SG is fixed at 1.010 seen in chronic renal failure
		b. SG >1.030 hyperosmolar urine, seen in diabetes mellitus, severe dehydration, adrenal insufficiency and nephrotic syndrome
		c. SG <1.008 hypos molar urine, seen in diabetes insipidus, compulsive polydipsia

Pathological Chemical Constituents Commonly seen in Urine

Abnormal constituents	Pathological condition
1. Glucose	a. Diabetes mellitus
2. Albumin	a. Nephrotic syndrome
	b. Eclampsia and pre-eclampsia
	c. Heart failure
	d. UTI
	e. Inflammatory kidney diseases
3. Blood	a. UTI
	b. Kidney stones
	c. Tumors related to renal system
	d. Hemoglobinopathies
4. Bile salt	a. Obstructive jaundice
5. Bile pigments	a. Obstructive jaundice
6. Urobilinogen	a. Obstructive jaundice
7. Pentose	a. Essential pentosuria
8. Bence-Jones protein	a. Multiple myeloma
9. Ketone bodies	a. Diabetic ketoacidosis
	b. Starvation
	c. Hyperemesis gravidarum

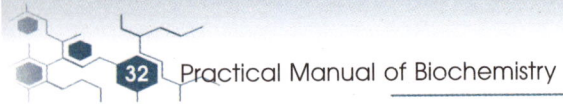

Abnormal Constituents of Urine (Pathological Urine)

Test	Principle	Observation		Inference
Reducing sugar: Benedict test Reagents: Sodium citrate + sodium carbonate + copper sulphate **Procedure:** 5 ml reagent + 7–8 drop of urine sample + boil 2–3 min + cool	Reducing sugars have free aldehyde or ketone group, which reduces metallic ions. Benedict reagent has cupric ion which is reduced to cuprous ion	color Green yellow orange Brick red blue (Fig. 4.6)	Con 0.5–1% 1–1.5% 1.5–2% >2% No sugar	Presence of reducing sugar
Protein heat coagulation test-procedure: Fill ¾ test tube with sample + heat upper part + coagulum formed + add 2–3% CH_3COOH If coagulum is dissolves, indicate presence of phosphate	Denaturation of protein by heat	Coagulum is formed at upper part (Fig. 4.8a)		Presence of protein
Heller's test-reagents: HNO_3 **Procedure:** 3 ml of sample + add 3–4 ml of HNO_3 along the side wall of tube	Nitric acid cause precipitation of protein	White ring formed at junction of two liquid (Fig. 4.8b)		Protein present
Bence Jones proteins: Procedure: Heat 40–60°C– ppt + heat 100°C– dissolve ppt + cool again reapper		Heat–ppt disappear cool– reappear		Presence of Bence Jones proteins
Ketone bodies: Rothera's nitroprusside test reagents: Ammonium sulfate, sodium nitroprusside, liquor ammonia **Procedure:** 5 ml urine saturate with ammonium sulfate + sodium nitroprusside + shake + liquor ammonia side of tube	Ketone bodies form a purple colored complex with sodium nitroprusside in alkaline medium. β-hydroxybutyrate does not give this test	Purple ring formed at the junction of two liquid (Fig. 4.7)		Presence of ketone bodies
Bile salt Hay's sulfur test reagents—sulfur powder Procedure: 4–5 ml of sample in tube + add pinch of sulfur powder on surface	Bile salt reduces the surface tension of water	Sulfur powder sinks towards bottom (Figs 4.9a, and b)		Presence of bile salts
Bile pigments Fouchet's test reagent: ($FeCl_3$+TCA) 6 ml $BaCl_2$ add 10–11 ml urine sample + filter Add 1–2 drop of reagent	$BaCl_2$ reacts with sulfur to form barium sulfate	Green blue color appear		Presence of bilirubin
Urobilinogen Ehrlich's test-reagent: (p-dimethyl-aminobenzaldehyde) **Procedure:** 5–6 ml urine + 5 ml of reagent + wait 8–10 min + add 10 ml saturated sodium acetate	Urobilinogen in acidic medium react with Ehrlich's reagent to form colored compound	Pink, red color		Presence of urobilinogen
Blood pigment benzidine test-reagents: H_2O_2 **Procedure:** 2–3 drop saturate benzidine solution + add 3 ml sample + 4 drop H_2O_2	Peroxidase like activity of hemoglobin $H_2O_2 \rightarrow H_2O + O$ (O) oxidizes the benzidine to form blue/green colored oxidized product	Blue green color develop		Presence of blood pigment

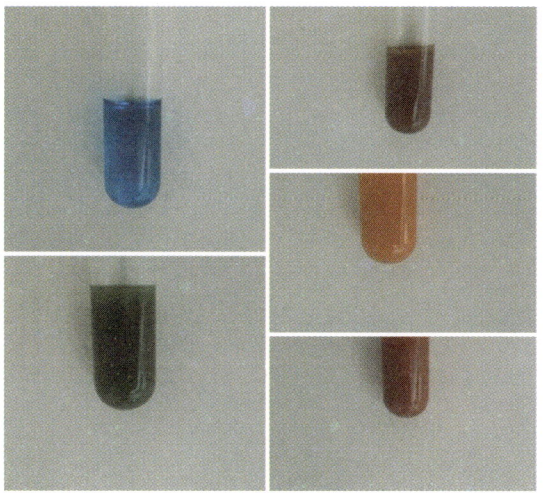

Fig. 4.6: Benedict's test

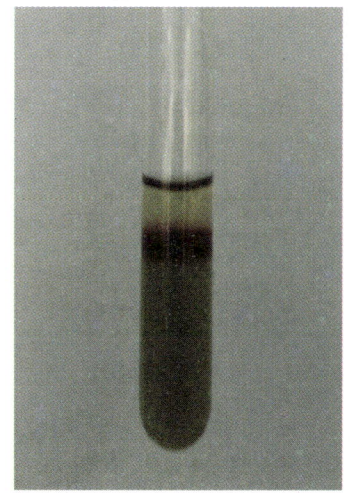

Fig. 4.7: Rothera's test

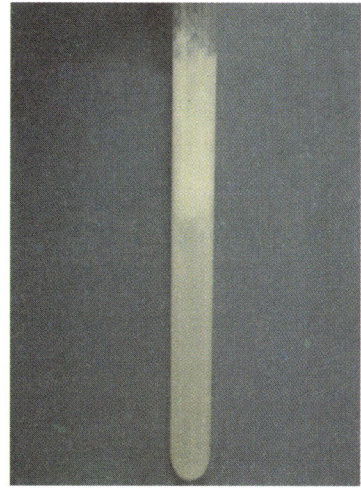

Fig. 4.8a: Heat coagulation test

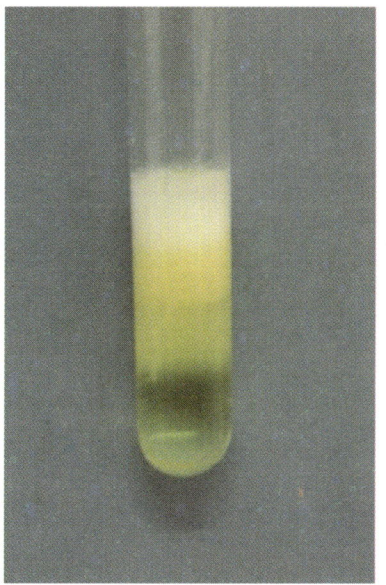

Fig. 4.8b: Heller's nitric acid test

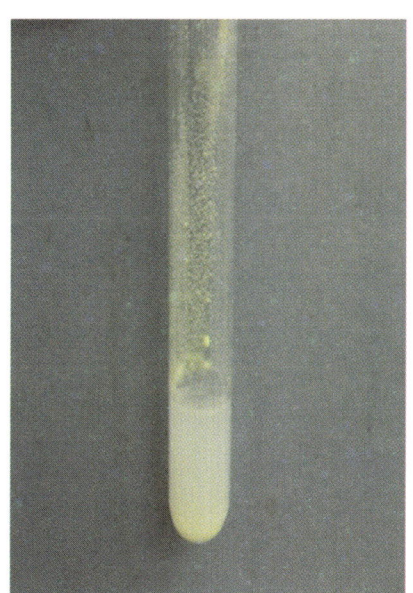

Fig. 4.9a: Hay sulfur test

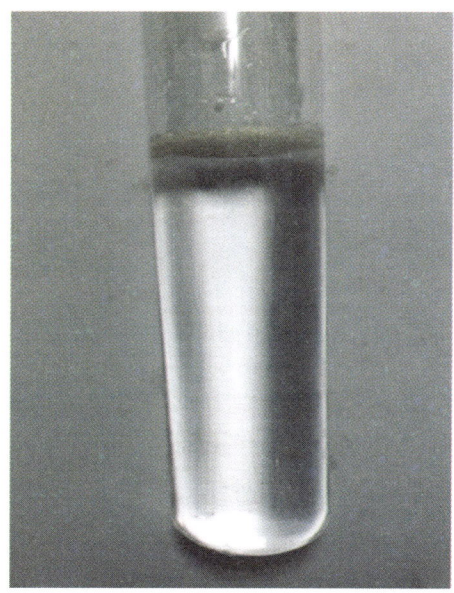

Fig. 4.9b: Control hay sulfur test

VIVA VOCE

Q1. What is the specific gravity for normal urine?

Ans. 1.010–1.025

Q2. How specific gravity changes in diabetes insipidus?

Ans. It is low, fixed below 1.010.

Q3. In which conditions color of urine sample can be changed?

Ans. Jaundice-deep yellow, red—hemoglobinuria, blood, dark amber—vitamin B complex therapy.

Q4. Name of ketone bodies.

Ans. Acetone, acetoacetate, beta hydroxy butyric acid.

Q5. When ketone bodies appear in urine?

Ans. Uncontrolled diabetes mellitus, severe starvation.

Q6. Write common causes for proteinuria.

Ans. Nephrotic syndrome, diabetic nephropathy, renal failure, CHD.

Q7. Commonly which protein come into urine?

Ans. Albumin.

Q8. Name of bile salts.

Ans. Sodium and potassium cholic and chenodeoxycholic acid.

Q9. Name of bile pigments.

Ans. Bilirubin, billiverdin.

Q10. Presence of Bence Jones protein in urine indicate.......

Ans. Multiple myeloma.

Q11. Name few conditions where specific gravity of urine increases.

Ans. Diabetes mellitus, proteinuria, presence of ketone bodies in urine.

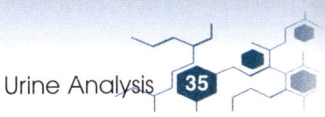

Quantitative Analysis

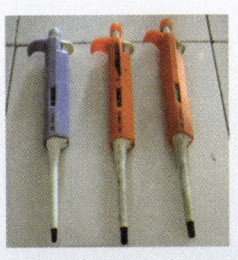
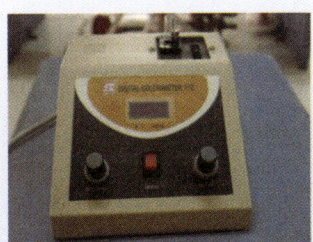
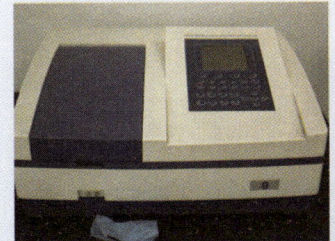
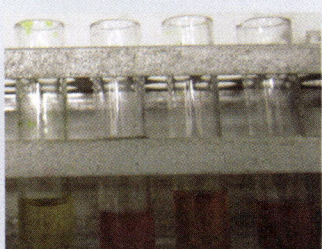

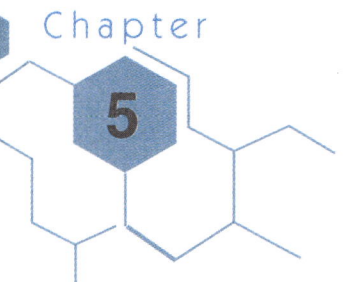
Colorimeter

The instrument commonly used is colorimetry which uses the basic principle of photometer. Colorless compounds are converted into colored compounds using chemical reactions. It uses light only in the visible region (400–760 nm).

Principle of colorimetry: It obeys beer lambert law. It is a combination of two laws.

Beer's law: Beer's law states that the absorption of light is directly proportional to the concentration of substance.

$$A \alpha C$$

C—concentration of substance
A—absorbance

Lambert's law: This law states that the absorption of light is directly proportional to the path length travelled by the light.

$$A \alpha t$$

$A = KCt$
$Log1/T = KCt$

K = constant

Log1/T = optical density (**OD**) or tranmittance

A—Absorbance

C—Concentration of substance

Parts of Colorimeter

1. Source of light: Tungsten lamp

2. Filter: Visible range (400–760 nm)

3. Cuvette: Plain tube

4. Photocell: Convert light energy into electrical energy

$$Light\ energy \rightarrow Electrical\ energy$$

5. Measuring device: Galvanometer it can read transmittance and absorbance.

Wavelength	Region	Color/filter
<380	U.V	Not visible
380–440	Visible	Violet (green-yellow)
440–500	Visible	Blue (yellow)
500–580	Visible	Green (red)
580–600	Visible	Yellow (blue)
600–620	Visible	Orange (green blue)
620–750	Visible	Red (green)
>750	IR	Not visible

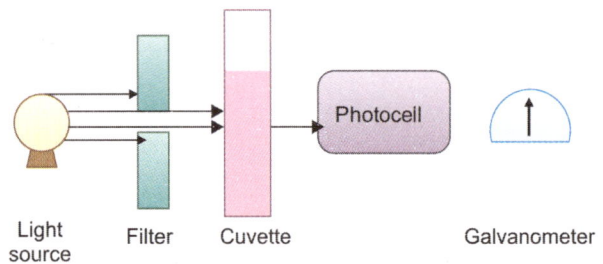

Fig. 5.1: Parts of colorimeter (*Courtesy:* Dr Sohil)

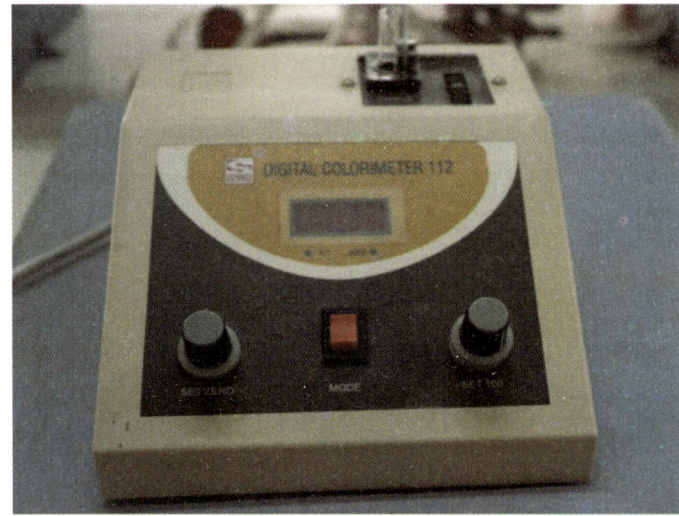

Fig. 5.2: Instrument

Calculation

$$\text{conc of substance} = \frac{\text{OD of test}}{\text{OD of std}} \times \frac{\text{Vol of standard}}{\text{Vol of serum/sample}} \times \text{conc of std}$$

SPECTROPHOTOMETER

More sensitive and accurate than colorimeter

Works on Beer Lambert's law.

It covers UV, visible and IR region.

Range	Region
200–400 nm	UV
400–700 nm	Visible
>700 nm	IR

Light source: Quartz and deuterium lamp

Cuvette: Quartz

Filter: Prism

Auto Analyzer

- Fully automatic device to measure the absorbance of substance.
- It display results on screen and can also be printed by printer.

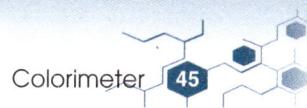

Principle

- It covers Beer Lambert's law in chemistry.
- In immunochemistry (endocrinology) it follows the principle of chemilumnisence (ECLIA).

Component

- Spectrophotometer/colorimeter component
- Sample tray
- Reagent tray
- Probes
- Cuvette
- Heating and cooling device
- Waste
- Internal and external computer (display)
- Barcode reader
- Printer.

VIVA VOCE

Q1. Difference between colorimeter and spectrophotometer.

Ans.

Spectrophotometer	Colorimeter
More accurate	Less accurate
More sensitive	Less sensitive
Filter: prism	Filter: visible (400–700)
Region: UV, visible, IR	Region: visible
Cuvette: Quartz	Cuvette: plain tube
Light source: Quartz, deuterium lamp	Light source: Tungsten lamp

Q2. What is OD?

Ans. 1/T, negative logarithm of transmittance.

Q3. What is the range of OD in colorimeter?

Ans. 0–2.

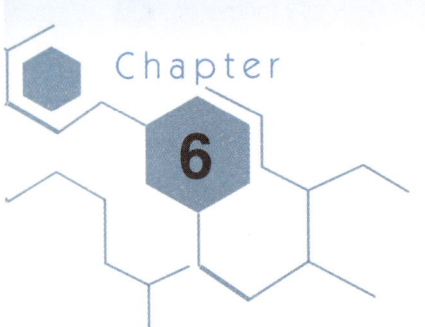

Estimation of Blood Glucose

Introduction: Estimation of blood glucose use for routine diagnosis of diabetes mellitus hyperglycemia.

Methods of Estimation of Glucose

Enzymatic method: GOD-POD method.

Hexokinase Method

Method based on reducing property: Folin and Wu method.

Nelson and somogyi method.

Asatoor and king method.

Ortho-toludine method.

Aim: Estimation of blood glucose by colorimeter.

Principle: GOD-POD (End point method glucose oxidase-peroxidase method)

$$\text{Glucose} + O_2 \xrightarrow{\text{Glucose oxidase}} \text{Gluconic acid} + H_2O_2$$

$$H_2O_2 + \text{phenol} + \text{4-aminoantipyrine} \xrightarrow{\text{Peroxidase}} \text{Red quinine dye} + H_2O$$

Procedure: Take 1 ml reagent in tube

Add 10 µl serum

↓

Mix well and incubate for 10 min at 37°C

↓

Read at 520 nm

Observation Table

	Blank	Standard	Test
Reagent	1 ml	1 ml	1 ml
Standard	–	10 µl	–
Serum	–	–	10 µl

Calculation

Results: ....

Normal range of blood glucose:

Fasting blood glucose—70–110 mg/dl.

Random blood glucose—70–130 mg/dl.

Postprandial (pp) glucose—70–140 mg/dl.

Interpretation

Conditions when blood glucose elevated	Hyperglycemia
	Fasting >110 mg/dl
	Pp >140 mg/dl
	1. Hyperactivity of endocrine gland (thyroid, pituitary and adrenal)
	2. Emotional stress
	3. Disease of pancreas
	4. Diabetes mellitus
Conditions when blood glucose decreased	Hypoglycemia
	Fasting <60 mg/dl
	1. Insulinoma
	2. Over dose of insulin
	3. Prolong starvation
	4. Hypoactivity of adrenal gland

VIVA VOCE

Q1. Which vial is used for glucose estimation?

Ans. Sodium fluoride.

Q2. Name of method for glucose estimation.

Ans. GOD-POD.

Q3. What is the range for fasting and PP glucose?

Ans. F-70–110 mg/dl.
PP up to 140 mg/dl.

Q4. What are the causes of hyperglycemia?

Ans. DM, hyperactivity of adrenal and pituitary.

Q5. What are the causes of hypoglycemia?

Ans. Over dose of insulin, prolonged starvation.

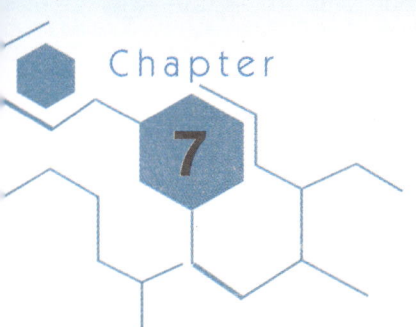

Kidney Function Test

A. ESTIMATION OF BLOOD UREA

INTRODUCTION

Urea is the end product of protein metabolism. Breakdown of protein forms amino acids, deamination of amino acids form NH_3. NH_3 is converted into urea in liver and kidney eliminates it in urine.

Methods of Urea Estimation

1. Berthelot method (phenol hypochlorite method).
2. Diacetyl monoxime (DAM) method.
3. Urease method.
4. Nesslerization method.

Aim: Estimation of blood urea by Berthelot method.

Principle: Urease act on urea to liberate NH_3, which combines with phenol and hypochlorite to form blue green color complex. The intensity of color is measured at 580 nm.

$$NH_3 + Phenol + Hypochlorite \xrightarrow{\text{Nitroprusside (alk med)}} Indo\ phenol\ (Blue\ green\ complex)$$

Procedure

	Blank	Test	Standard
Reagent 1	1 ml	1 ml	1 ml
Distilled water	10 µl	–	–
Urea standard	–	–	10 µl
Serum	–	10 µl	–
	Incubate for 5 mins		
Reagent 2	1 ml	1 ml	1 ml

Incubate for 10 mins. Read at 580 nm.

Calculation

$$\frac{\text{OD of test}}{\text{OD of std}} \times \frac{\text{Amt of std}}{\text{Volume of std}} \times 100$$

Results ....

Interpretation

Normal blood urea = 10– 40 mg/dl.
Normal urine urea = 23–30 g/day.
Normal blood urea nitrogen (BUN) = 7–25 mg/dl
(1 mg of BUN = 2.14 mg of urea).

Elevated Levels of Urea are seen in

Prerenal	1. Congestive heart failure 2. Shock and hemorrhage 3. Salt and water depletion 4. Dehydration due to vomiting and diarrhea 5. Ulcerative colitis 6. Pyloric stenosis with severe vomiting 7. Intestinal obstruction 8. Burns
Renal	1. Acute glomerulonephritis 2. Nephrotic syndrome 3. Malignant nephrosclerosis 4. Chronic pylonephritis 5. Renal tuberculosis 6. Mercurial poisoning
Postrenal	1. Prostate hypertrophy and cancer 2. Stone in urinary tract 3. Stricture of urethra 4. Tumor of bladder

Decrease urea levels are seen in:

1. Sever liver disease.
2. Cancer of liver.

Physiological variations are seen:

1. Pregnancy due to hemodilution.
2. Low in females.
3. Varies with amount of protein in diet.

Urea clearance:

Clearance is defined as volume of plasma cleared of a substance in one minute by kidney.
It is the measure of glomerular function of kidney.
Expressed in ml/min

$$C = \frac{U \times V}{P}$$

U = concentration of substance in urine.
V = volume of urine excreted per min.
P = concentration of substance in plasma.

Urea clearance depends on flow of urine.

When flow of urine is >2 ml/minute clearance is 60–95 ml/minute (average = 75 ml/min), it is called maximum clearance.

When urine flow is <2 ml/minute clearance is 40–65 ml/minute (54 ml/min), it is called standard clearance.

If urea clearance is

Urea clearance	Renal impairment
70%	Normal
40–70%	Mild impairment
20–40%	Moderate impairment
<20%	Severe impairment

Urea clearance is not a better index of glomerular function as only 10% of urea is excreted.

VIVA VOCE

Q1. What is normal level of urea in blood?

Ans. 20–40 mg/dl.

Q2. What are the causes of increased blood urea level?

Ans. Prerenal, renal, postrenal.

Q3. Explain few prerenal conditions.

Ans. Fever, CHD, dehydration.

Q4. Explain renal and postrenal conditions.

Ans. See on last page.

Q5. Conditions when blood urea level decreased?

Ans. Cirrhosis of liver.

B. ESTIMATION OF SERUM CREATININE

INTRODUCTION

Creatine is synthesized in liver from glycine, arginine and methionine. It then reaches muscle via blood. Creatine kinase converts creatine into creatine phosphate. Creatine phosphate acts as a storage form of ATP. Creatinine is formed spontaneously and non-enzymatically from creatine phosphate at the rate of 2% of total body creatine per day.

Amount excreted in urine remain constant for a given person and depends only on muscle mass and is independent of protein in diet. Therefore, serum creatinine is a better index of renal function.

Methods of Creatinine Estimation

1. Jaffe's reaction.

2. Nitroprusside test.

Aim: Estimation of serum creatinine by Jaffe's method.

Principle: Creatinine reacts with picric acid in alkaline medium to form orange red creatinine picrate. The intensity is measured at 520 nm.

Procedure

	Blank	Standard	Test
Jaffe's reagent	1 ml	1 ml	1 ml
Distilled water	100 μl	–	–
Standard	–	100 μl	–
Serum	–	–	100 μl

Mix well and allow stand for 15 minutes and read at 520 nm.

Calculation

$$C = \frac{\text{OD of test}}{\text{OD of std}} \times \frac{\text{Amt of std}}{\text{Volume of std}} \times 100$$

Results ....

Interpretation

Normal range

Males: 0.7–1.4 mg/dl.

Females: 0.6–1.2 mg/dl.

Elevated levels are seen in:

1. Renal failure and other renal diseases.

2. Early stages of muscular dystrophy/poliomyelitis.

Creatinine Clearance

Clearance is defined as volume of plasma cleared of creatinine in one minute by kidney.

It is the measure of glomerular function of kidney.

Expressed in ml/min

$$C = \frac{U \times V}{P}$$

U = concentration of substance in urine.

V = volume of urine excreted per minute.

P = concentration of substance in plasma.

Cretinine is negligibly reabsorb and is not secreted by renal tubules; therefore, its clearance is almost similar to GFR.

Normal creatinine clearance:

Males: 94–140 ml/minute.

Females: 72–110 ml/minute.

VIVA VOCE

Q1. What is the normal serum creatinine level?

Ans. Males: 0.7– 1.5 Mg/dl.
Females: 0.4–1.2 mg/dl.

Q2. Amino acids involved in creatinine synthesis.

Ans. Glycine, arginine, methionine.

Q3. Why is estimation of serum creatinine a better index of KFT than blood urea?

Ans. Its level depends on glomerular filtration not affected by diet and other factors.

Q4. What is the normal daily excretion of creatinine in urine?

Ans. 1–2 gm/day.

Q5. Name of method for creatinine estimation?

Ans. Jaffe's method.

C. ESTIMATION OF SERUM URIC ACID

INTRODUCTION

Uric acid is the end product of purines metabolism. It is completely reabsorbed in proximal convoluted tubules and then secreted into distal convoluted tubules. It is partly reabsorbed and partly excreted in urine.

Methods of Uric Acid Estimation

1. Phosphotungstic acid method.
2. Uricase method.
3. High pressure liquid chromatography method.

Aim: Estimation of blood uric acid level by uricase method.

Principle: Uricase enzyme act on uric acid to liberate H_2O_2. H_2O_2 reacts with 4-aminophenazone (4AP) and 2,4dichlorophenol sulfonate (DCPS) in presence of peroxidase to form a red colored complex quinoneimine compound.

$$\text{Uric acid} + 2H_2O + O_2 \xrightarrow{\text{Uricase}} \text{Allantoin} + CO_2 + H_2O_2$$

$$2H_2O_2 + 4AP + DCPS \xrightarrow{\text{POD}} \text{Quinoneimine} + 4H_2O$$

Intensity of color is directly proportional to the concentration of uric acid.

Procedure

	Blank	Standard	Test
Working reagent	1 ml	1 ml	1 ml
Standard	–	25 µl	–
Serum	–	–	25 µl
Distilled water	25 µl	–	–

Mix and incubate for 3 minutes at 37°C and read at 650°C.

Calculation

$$\text{conc of uric acid} = \frac{\text{OD of test}}{\text{OD of std}} \times \frac{\text{Vol of standard}}{\text{Vol of serum/sample}} \times \text{conc of std}$$

Results ....

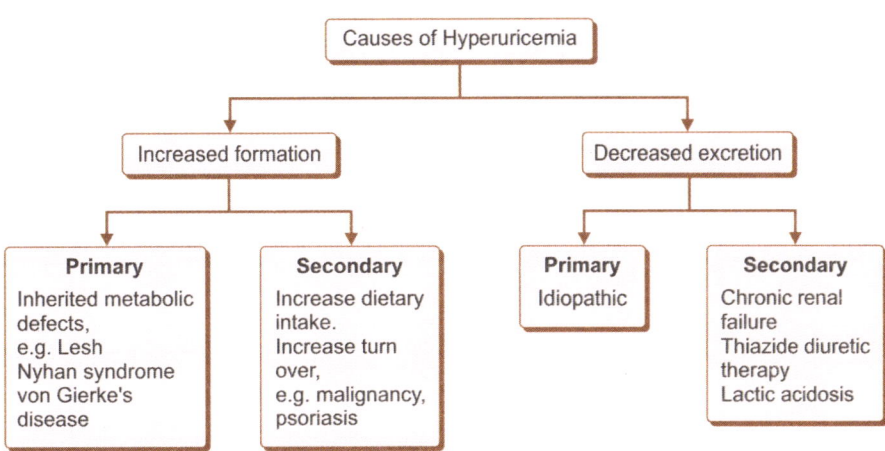

Interpretation

Normal range

Males: 4.5–7.5 mg/dl.

Females: 2.3–6.5 mg/dl.

Causes of Hyperuricemia

Hyporuricemia: When uric acid concentration <2 mg/dl. It is a rare condition seen in:

1. Severe liver disease, purine synthesis decreases.
2. Defective renal tubular reabsorption.

VIVA VOCE

Q1. What is the normal level of uric acid?

Ans. 2–7 mg/dl.

Q2. What are the causes of hyperuricemia?

Ans. Renal failure, leukemia, HGPRTase deficiency.

Q3. Is there any correlation between cancer and uric acid?

Ans. Yes, hyperuricemia, because of increased cell growth, increase breakdown of purines cause to Gout.

Q4. How alcohol affect uric acid level?

Ans. Alcohol increase NADH it is promote formation of monosodium urate, that is less soluble.

Q5. What is tophi?

Ans. Deposition of uric acid crystals in joints or skin or cartilage. Most common site of deposition of crystal in big toe.

Q6. Why do cancer patients have high levels of uric acid?

Ans. Cancer patients have high cell turnover this causes increase breakdown of purine and hence increase formation of uric acid.

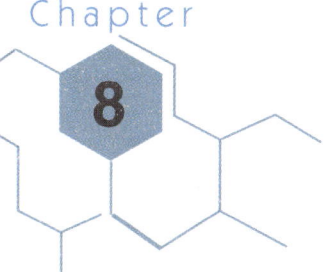

Chapter

8

Lipidogram

A. ESTIMATION OF TOTAL CHOLESTEROL

INTRODUCTION

Cholesterol is one of the causative factors of heart disease, thrombosis, cerebral hemorrhage.

Cholesterol
- Free 30%
- Estrified 70%

Total plasma lipids are in serum 400–600 mg/dl

Total cholesterol	200–250 mg/dl
Serum triglycerides	25–170 mg/dl
Serum HDL—cholesterol	35–60 mg/dl
Serum LDL—cholesterol	Up to 150 mg/dl
Serum VLDL—cholesterol	20–35 mg/dl

Aim: Estimation of total cholesterol by colorimetry.

Methods: CHOD-POD method.

Libermann-Burchard's method.

ZAK's method.

Sackets's method.

Kim and goldberg.

Salkowski's method.

Principle: (CHOD-POD method)

Cholesterol ester $+ H_2O \rightarrow$ Cholesterol + FFA

Cholesterol + $O_2 \rightarrow$ Cholesterol + H_2O_2

H_2O_2 + phenol + 4-aminoantipyrine $\rightarrow$ quinoneimine + H_2O
(Red/pink dye)

Procedure

Take 1 ml reagent in tube
↓
Add 20 µl serum
↓
Mix well and incubate at room temperature for 10 minutes AT 37°C
↓
Read at 520 nm

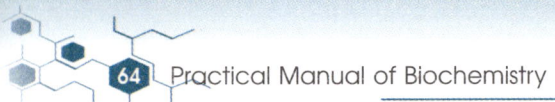

Observation Table

	Blank	Standard	Test
Reagent	1 ml	1 ml	1 ml
Standard	–	20 µl	–
Serum	–	–	20 µl

Calculation

$$\frac{\text{OD of test}}{\text{OD of standard}} \times \text{conc of standard}$$

Results: ....

Normal range of cholesterol in blood 200–250 mg/dl.

Interpretation

Hypocholestremia	1. Hyperthyroidism
	2. Abetalipoproteinemia
Hypercholestremia	1. Hypothyroidism
	2. von-Gierke's disease
	3. Nephrotic syndrome
	4. Alcohol intake
	5. Obstructive jaundice
	6. Diabetes mellitus

VIVA VOCE

Q1 What is the normal blood cholesterol range?

Ans. 150–250 mg/dl.

Q2. Number of carbon atom present in cholesterol structure.

Ans. 27.

Q3. Name of products formed by the degrading of cholesterol.

Ans. Bile acids, vitamin D, steroid hormones.

Q4. Name of dietary sources for cholesterol.

Ans. Milk, egg, meat.

Q5. Condition for Hypo- and hyper-cholesterolemia

Ans. See on last page.

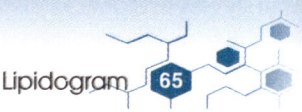

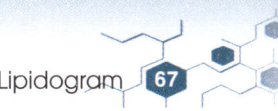

B. ESTIMATION OF TRIGLYCERIDES (TG)

INTRODUCTION

TG estimation is very important for diagnosis and management of hyperlipidemias, nephrosis, diabetes mellitus, and endocrine disorders.

Aim: Estimation of triglycerides by colorimetric method.

Method: Trinder method.

Principle

$$\text{Triglycerides} + H_2O \xrightarrow{\text{Lipase}} \text{Glycerol} + FFA$$

$$\text{Glycerol} + ATP \xrightarrow{\text{Glycerol kinase}} \text{Glycerol 3-PO}_4 + ADP$$

$$\text{Glycerol 3PO}_4 + O_2 \xrightarrow{\text{Oxidase}} DHAP + H_2O_2$$

$$H_2O_2 + \text{4-aminoantipyrine} + \text{phenol} \xrightarrow{\text{Peroxidase}} \text{Quinoneimine dye}$$
$$\text{(Red/pink color)}$$

Procedure

Take 1 ml reagent in tube
↓
Add 10 µl serum
↓
Mix well and incubate at room temperature for 10 minutes (37°C)
↓
Read at 520 nm

Observation Table

	Blank	*Standard*	*Test*
Reagent	1 ml	1 ml	1 ml
Standard	–	10 µl	–
Serum	–	–	10 µl

Calculation

$$\frac{\text{OD of test}}{\text{OD of standard}} \times \text{conc of standard}$$

Results:.................

Normal range of TG in blood 25–170 mg/dl.

Interpretation

TG level ↑	1. Diabetes mellitus
	2. Nephrosis
	3. Hypothyroidism
	4. Pregnancy
	5. Alcoholism
	6. Atherosclerosis
	7. Ischemic heart disease
	8. Intake of OCPs

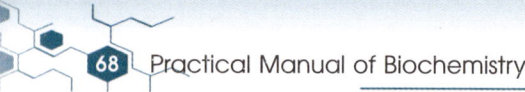

VIVA VOCE

Q1. What is the normal range of TG in serum?

Ans. 25–170 mg/dl.

Q2. Conditions when increases serum TG levels ?

Ans. See on last page.

Q3. Name of method for TG estimation.

Ans. Trinder method.

Q4. Which color filter use for TG estimation?

Ans. 520 nm green filter.

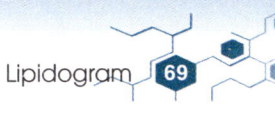

C. HDL ESTIMATION IN LIPIDOGRAM

INTRODUCTION

HDL cholesterol is good cholesterol its action is cardioprotective because it transport cholesterol from peripheral tissue to liver (reverse transport of cholesterol).

Aim: Estimation of HDL by colorimetry.

Method: Phosphotungstic acid method.

Principle: Serum phosphotungstate → HDL + (LDL + VLDL + Chylomicrons).

Procedure: Precipitation.

Pipette	Volume
Test	250 µl
Precipitating reagent	500 µl

Mixing and stand for 10 minutes at room temperature centrifuge at 4000 rpm for 10 minutes supernatant

↓

Take 1 ml reagent (cholesterol)

↓

Add 50 µl serum

(**supernatant**)

↓

Mix well and incubate 10 min at 37°C

↓

Read at 505 nm

Observation Table

	Blank	Standard	Test
Reagent	1 ml	1 ml	1 ml
Standard	–	50 µl	–
Serum (supernatant)	–	–	50 µl

Calculation

$$\frac{\text{OD of test}}{\text{OD of standard}} \times \text{conc of standard}$$

Results: ....

Normal range of HDL in male 30–65 mg/dl.

Normal range of HDL in female 30–80 mg/dl.

Interpretation

HDL level ↓	Atherosclerosis
	Smoking
	Alcoholism
	Myocardial infraction
	Coronary heart disease

LdL-c and VLDL estimation (Friedewald's equation)

Total cholesterol = VLDL + HDL + LDL

LDL = Total cholesterol-(TG/5-HDL)

VLDL = TG/5

VIVA VOCE

Q1. What is the normal HDL level in serum?

Ans. 30–70 mg/dl.

Q2. Name of the enzyme which take part in reverse cholesterol transport?

Ans. LCAT.

Q3. Why HDL is known as good cholesterol?

Ans. Because of reverse cholesterol transport, it esterifies cholesterol and transfer to liver.

Q4. Name of Apo protein present in HDL.

Ans. Apo A, Apo E, Apo CII.

Q5. How to calculate VLDL?

Ans. TG/5.

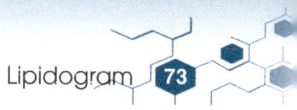

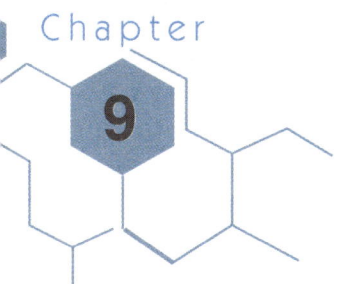

Liver Function Test

Liver function test is routinely done to assess the function of the liver.

The test routinely done in LFT are:

1. Total bilirubin
2. Direct bilirubin
3. Indirect bilirubin
4. Total protein
5. Albumin
6. Globulin
7. SGOT
8. SGPT
9. Alkaline phosphatase.

ESTIMATION OF BILIRUBIN TOTAL/DIRECT/INDIRECT

INTRODUCTION

Bilirubin is a catabolic product of heme metabolism. Conjugation of bilirubin occurs in liver. Estimation of bilirubin is very important for diagnosis of liver disease.

Aim: Estimation of bilirubin (total/direct/indirect).

Method: Diazo method.

Principle

Bilirubin + diazotized sulphanilic acid $\rightarrow$ azobilirubin (pink).

Bilirubin direct—directly react in acidic medium (water soluble).

Indirect bilirubin—Indirect bilirubin solubilised after addition of surfactant.

Procedure

Total Bilirubin Reagent (R_1)

Surfactant	1%
HCl	100 mmol/L
Sulphanilic acid	5 mmol/L

Direct Bilirubin Reagent (R_2)

Sulphanilic acid	10 mmol/L
HCl	100 mmol/L

Reagent (R_3): Sodium nitrite 144 mmol/L.

Reagent Preparation

Test	Volume of working reagent	Add		
		R1	R2	R3
Bilirubin total	10 ml	10 ml		0.2 ml
Bilirubin direct	10 ml		10 ml	0.1 ml

Keep the reagent 3 vial plugged after use.

Observation Table

Total Bilirubin/Direct Bilirubin

Pipette in to test tube	Blank	Standard	Test
Working reagent	500 µl	500 µl	500 µl
DW	25 µl		
Standard		25 µl	
Test			**25 µl**

Mix well incubate for 5 minutes at 37°C for total bilirubin and direct bilirubin. And read at 540–630 nm.

Calculation

$$\frac{\text{OD of test}}{\text{OD of standard}} \times \text{conc of standard}$$

Normal range of total bilirubin—0.2–1 mg/dl.
Indirect bilirubin 0.2–0.6 mg/dl.
Direct bilirubin 0.2–0.4 mg/dl.

Results. ....

Interpretation

Indirect bilirubin	• Hemolytic Jaundice
	• Gilbert syndrome
	• Neonates
	• Crigller—Najjar type I
	• Crigller—Najjar type II
Direct bilirubin	• Obstructive jaundice
	• Hepatocellular jaundice
	• Rotor syndrome
	• Dubin-Johnson syndrome

ESTIMATION OF TOTAL PROTEIN

INTRODUCTION

Protein is the polymer of L-α amino acid. Blood contain large number of protein they perform so many functions. Most of enzymes, hormones, and clotting factors are protein in nature.

Methods of Estimation of Protein

- Biuret method
- Lowry method
- Dye-binding method
- Turbidimetric method
- Nephelometric method
- Kjeldahl's method.

Aim: Estimation of protein by colorimeter.

Method: Biuret method.

Principle: All compounds contain minimum two peptide linkage in alkaline medium peptide bond react with biuret reagent. Cupric ion forms chelate with peptide bond and form purple–violet color complex.

Procedure

Take 1 ml reagent in tube

↓

Add 20 µl serum

↓

Mix well and incubate 10 min at 37°C

↓

Read at 540 nm

Observation Table

	Blank	Standard	Test
Reagent	1 ml	1 ml	1 ml
Standard	–	20 µl	–
Serum	–	–	20 µl

Calculation

$$\frac{\text{OD of test}}{\text{OD of standard}} \times \text{conc of standard}$$

Results. ....

Normal range of blood protein:

Total protein: 6–8 g/dl.

Serum albumin: 3.5–5.5 g/dl.

Serum globulin: 2.5–3.5 g/dl.

A/G ratio: 1.4–1.15 g/dl.

Interpretation

Conditions when serum protein elevated	Hyperproteinemia 1. Dehydration
Conditions when serum protein decreased	Hyperproteinemia 1. Malnutrition 2. Liver disease 3. Prolong starvation 4. Nephrotic syndrome

VIVA VOCE

Q1. Bilirubin is the catabolic end product of which substance?

Ans. By catabolism of heme.

Q2. Write names of water soluble and insoluble bilirubin.

Ans. Conjugated is water soluble and unconjugated is insoluble in water.

Q3. How to define jaundice?

Ans. Yellow discoloration of skin, conjunctiva, mucosa and increase level of bilirubin is known as jaundice.

Q4. Types of jaundice?

Ans. Prehepatic, hepatic, posthepatic.

Q5. Causes of prehepatic, hepatic and posthepatic jaundice.

Ans. Prehepatic—G6PD deficiency, blood transfusion mismatch.
Hepatic—Alcohol intake, hepatitis A, B, C, E, drug induced.
Posthepatic—Stone, cancer of head of pancrease.

ESTIMATION OF SERUM ALBUMIN

INTRODUCTION

Albumin is a major plasma protein perform so many function like transport, maintain colloid osmotic pressure, buffering action and nutritive so albumin act as complete protein. Synthesis of albumin occurs in liver.

Aim: Estimation of serum albumin by colorimeter.

Method: Bromocresol green (BCG).

Principle: Albumin binds with BCG and form blue green color complex.

$$BCG \text{ (undissociated form)} \longrightarrow BCG \text{ (dissociated form)}$$
$$\text{Yellow color} \qquad\qquad \text{blue color}$$

Procedure

Take 1 ml reagent in tube
↓
Add 10 µl serum
↓
Mix well and incubate 10 min at 37°C
↓
Read at 630 nm

Observation Table

	Blank	Standard	Test
Reagent	1 ml	1 ml	1 ml
Standard	–	10 µl	–
Serum	–	–	10 µl

Calculation

$$\text{conc of substance} = \frac{\text{OD of test}}{\text{OD of Std}} \times \frac{\text{Vol of standard}}{\text{Vol of serum/sample}} \times \text{conc of std}$$

Results: ....

Normal Range of Blood Protein

Total protein: 6–8 g/dl.

Serum albumin: 3.5–5.5 g/dl.

Serum globulin: 2.5–3.5 g/dl.

A/G ratio: 1.4–1.15 g/dl.

Interpretation

Conditions when serum albumin elevated	Hyperalbuminemia
	1. Dehydration
	2. Shock
	3. Hemoconcentration

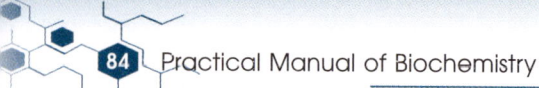

Conditions when serum albumin decreased	Hypoalbuminemia
	1. Malnutrition
	2. Liver disease
	3. Prolong starvation
	4. Nephrotic syndrome

Serum globulin = Total protein—serum albumin

A/G ratio = Serum albumin/serum globulin

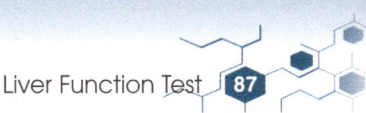

ESTIMATION OF SGOT/AST

INTRODUCTION

SGOT is a serum enzyme high concentration of SGOT found in liver, heart muscle.

Aim: Estimation of serum glutamate oxalotransaminase/aspartate aminotransferase (SGOT/AST).

Method: IFCC method (international federation of clinical chemistry).

Principle

$$\text{L-Aspartate + 2-oxoglutrate} \xrightarrow{\text{AST}} \text{Oxaloacetate + L-glutamate}$$

$$\text{Oxaloacetate + NADH} \xrightarrow{\text{MDH}} \text{L-Lactate + NAD}$$

$$\text{Sample pyruvate + NADH} \xrightarrow{\text{LDH}} \text{L-Lactate + NAD}$$

AST—Aspartate aminotransferase.

LDH—Lactate dehydrogenase.

MDH—Malate dehydrogenase.

Procedure

Pipette	Volumes
Working reagent	1000 µl
Test	100 µl

Mix well and aspirate.

Lagging time 60 sec.

Reading time 60 sec.

Read at 340 nm.

Calculation

$$IU/L = \frac{(\Delta A/\text{min}) \times TV \times 10^3}{SV \times \text{Absorption} \times P}$$

P: Cuvette light path = 1 cm.

TV: Total reagent volume in µl.

SV: Sample volume in µ.

Results: ....

Interpretation

Increased level of SGOT are seen in:

1. Heart diseases.
2. Myocardial infraction.
3. Liver diseases.

VIVA VOCE

Q1. Parameters included in LFT profile.

Ans. Bilirubin total, direct, indirect, total protein serum albumin, globulin, A/G ratio SGOT, SGPT, ALP.

Q2. Normal value of SGOT.

Ans. 10–45 IU/L.

Q3. Which enzymes increase in liver disease?

Ans. SGPT, SGOT.

Q4. Very high level of SGPT and SGOT are seen in:

Ans. Acute hepatitis, cardiac disease.

Q5. SGOT and SGPT are dependent on which coenzyme?

Ans. Pyridoxal phosphate (PLP).

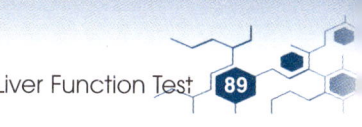

ESTIMATION OF SERUM SGPT/ALT

INTRODUCTION

SGPT is a serum enzyme high concentration of SGPT found in liver.

Aim: Estimation of serum glutamate pyruvate oxalotransaminase/Alanine transaminase (SGPT/ALT).

Method: IFCC method (international federation of clinical chemistry).

Principle

$$\text{L-alanine + 2-oxoglutrate} \xrightarrow{\text{ALT}} \text{pyruvate + L-glutamate}$$

$$\text{Pyruvate + NADH} \xrightarrow{\text{LDH}} \text{L-Lactate + NADH}$$

Procedure

Pipette	Volumes
Working reagent	1000 µl
Test	100 µl

Mix well and aspirate.

Lagging time—60 sec.

Reading time—60 sec.

Read at—340 nm.

Calculation

$$IU/L = \frac{(\Delta A/min) \times TV \times 10^3}{SV \times Absorption \times P}$$

P: Cuvette light path = 1 cm.

TV: Total reaction volume in µl.

SV: Sample volume in µ.

Results: ....

Interpretation

Increased level of SGPT are seen in

- Liver diseases
- Viral hepatitis
- Toxic hepatitis
- Liver cirrhosis
- Dengue.

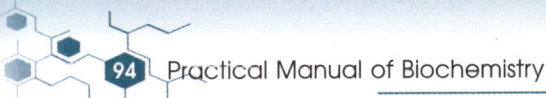

ESTIMATION OF ALKALINE PHOSPHATASE (ALP)

INTRODUCTION

ALP is produced by osteoblast of bone and associated with calcification of bone. ALP has different type of isoenzymes which are found in liver, bone, kidney, intestine and placenta.

Aim: Estimation of ALP by colorimeter.

Method: Kind and king method.

Principle

$$\text{Phenyl phosphate} \xrightarrow{\text{ALP}} \text{phenol} + p_i$$

$$\text{Phenol} + \text{4-aminoantipyrine} \xrightarrow{\text{Potassium ferricyanide}} \text{Orange/red color}$$

Procedure

	Blank	Standard	Control	Test
Reagent R1	500 µL	500 µL	500 µL	500 µL
DW	1500 µL	1500 µL	1500 µL	1500 µL

Mix well and incubate at 37°C for 3 minutes

Serum	–	–	–	50 µL
R3	–	50 µL	–	–

Mix well and incubate at 37°C for 15 minutes

R2	1000 µL	1000 µL	1000 µL	1000 µL
Serum	–	–	50 µL	–

Mix well read at 520 nm.

Calculation

$$= \frac{\text{OD of test} - \text{OD of control}}{\text{OD of standard} - \text{OD of blank}} \times \text{Conc of standard}$$

Results

Normal range of blood ALP: 29–130IU/L.
Increased levels are found in children.

Interpretation

Conditions when ALP elevated	Bone disease
	Obstructive jaundice
	Bone carcinoma
	Paget disease
	Liver cirrhosis
	Disease of intestinal tract
	Third trimester of pregnancy
	Growing children
Conditions when ALP decreased	Severe anemia
	Malnutrition

VIVA VOCE

Q1. Which enzyme increase in obstructive jaundice?
Ans. ALP.

Q2. What is the normal range of ALP in serum?
Ans. 29–129 IU/L.

Q3. How many isoenzymes of ALP are there?
Ans. Six isoenzymes (bone liver, placenta).

Q4. Which enzyme increase in bone disease?
Ans. ALP.

Q5. Various conditions where increased ALP levels are seen?
Ans. Hyperparathyroidism, disease of intestinal tract.

Q6. What is the normal range of ALP in children?
Ans. 104–345 U/L in 1–3 years.

Estimation of Blood Calcium

INTRODUCTION

99% of calcium is present in bones. In blood calcium is present in three forms:

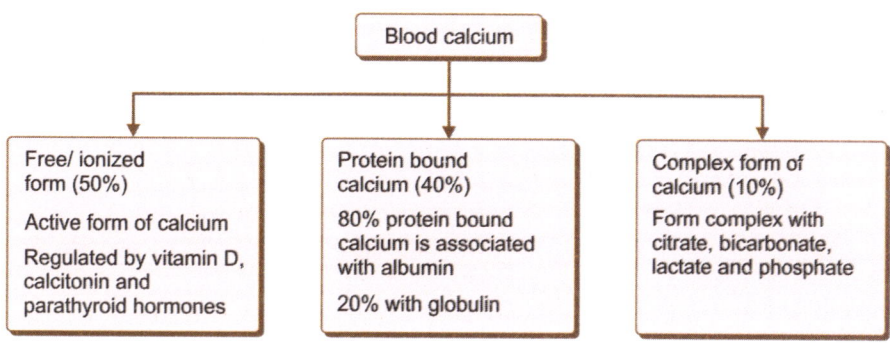

Regulation of Blood Calcium

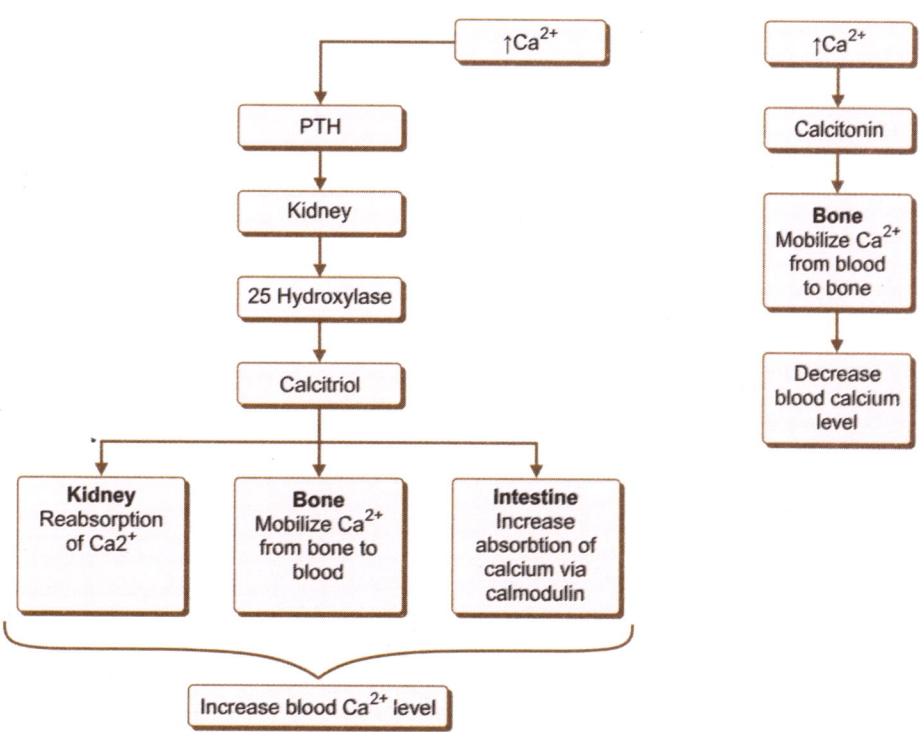

Role of Calcium

1. Present in bone along with phosphorus as hydroxyl apatite crystals.
2. Plays important role in blood coagulation cascade.
3. Muscle contraction.
4. Membrane permeability.
5. Neuromuscular transmission.
6. Act as secondary and tertiary messenger for hormone action.
7. Excitation of muscle and nerve tissue.

Methods of Calcium Estimation

1. o-Cresolphthalein complex-one (OCPC) method.
2. Arsenazo-III method.
3. Ion selective electrodes (ISE).
4. Atomic absorption spectrometry.
5. Titration method.

Aim: Estimation of blood calcium level Arsenazo III, end point method.

Principle: Calcium ions form violet complex with o-cresolphthalein complex-one in alkaline medium. Absorbance is measured at 570 nm. The intensity of color is directly proportional to the concentration of calcium ions.

Procedure

	Blank	Standard	Test
Working reagent	1 ml	1 ml	2.5 ml
Calcium standard	–	20 µl	–
Distilled water	20 µl	–	–
Serum	–	–	20 µl

Mix well then read at 650 nm filter.

Calculation

$$\frac{\text{OD of test}}{\text{OD of std}} \times \frac{\text{Volume of standard}}{\text{volume of serum}} \times 100$$

Result: ....

Interpretation

Normal range

Total calcium: 8–10 mg/dl.
Ionic calcium: 4.6–5.3 mg/dl.

Hypocalcemia	Hypercalcemia
1. Osteomalacia in adult	1. Hyperparathyroidism
2. Rickets in children	2. Hypervitaminosis D
3. Hypothyroidism	3. Bone cancer
4. Steatorrhea	4. Milk alkali syndrome
5. Pregnancy and lactation	5. Thyrotoxicosis
6. Nephritic syndrome	6. Multiple myeloma
7. Hepatocellular disease	7. Polycythemia vera
8. Hypomagnesemia	8. Sarcoidosis

VIVA VOCE

Q1. What is the normal range of serum calcium?

Ans. 9–11 mg/dl.

Q2. How many forms of calcium present in body?

Ans. Three forms. Ionized calcium, protein bound calcium, complexed calcium.

Q3. Write down regulation of calcium.

Ans. See on last page.

Q4. What is corrected calcium?

Ans. Serum calcium + 0.8 (4-serum albumin in gm%).

Q5. Write sources of calcium.

Ans. Milk, egg, dairy product.

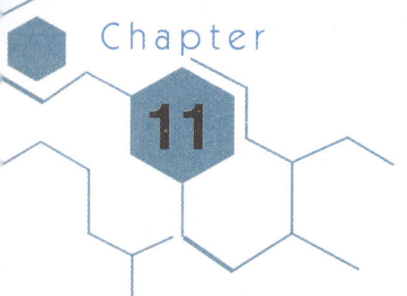

Estimation of Blood Phosphorus

INTRODUCTION

90% phosphorus is present in bones. In blood phosphorus is present in two forms:

1. **Organic form:** Phospholipids, glycerophosphate, nucleoside phosphate.

2. **Inorganic form:** Phosphates bound to various inorganic cations like Na^+, K^+, Ca^{2+}, etc.

Parathyroid hormone regulates the level of PO_4^{3-} in blood. PTH increases the excretion of PO_4^{3-} in urine and decreases its level. Vitamin D increases the level of PO_4^{3-} by increasing its absorption from intestine and reabsorption from renal tubules.

Methods of Estimation

1. Using reaction of phosphate ions with ammonium molybdate.

2. Vandate—molybdate method.

3. Enzymatic methods by monitoring the formation of NADPH, H_2O_2 and NADH.

Aim: Estimation of blood phosphate by ammonium molybdate method, end point.

Principle: Phosphate react with ammonium molybdate to form ammonium phospho molybdate which is reduced by reducer aminonaphthol sulphonic acid (ANSA) to form blue color.

Procedure

	Blank	Standard	Test
Reagent	1000 μl	1000 μl	1000 μl
Distilled water	20 μl	–	–
Standard	–	20 μl	–
Test	–	–	20 μl

Mix well and incubate at room temperature for 10 min, then read absorbance at 340 nm.

Calculations

$$\frac{\text{OD of test}}{\text{OD of std}} \times \frac{\text{Vol. of std}}{\text{Vol. of serum}} \times 100$$

Result: ....

Interpretation

Normal range

Adults: 2.5–4.5 mg/dl.

Children: 4–7 mg/dl.

Hyperphosphatemia	Hypophosphatemia
1. Renal failure	1. Hyperparathyroidism
2. Hypoparathyroidism	2. Fanconi's syndrome
3. Acromegaly	3. X-linked hypophosphatemia
4. Rhabdomyolysis	4. Malabsorption
5. Chemotherapy	5. Acidosis
6. Aggressive phosphate therapy	6. Respiratory alkalosis

VIVA VOCE

Q1. What is the normal range of serum phosphorus?

Ans. 3–5.5 mg/dl

Q2. Causes of decrease phosphorus level.

Ans. Hyperparathyroidism, diabetic coma, decrease renal tubular reabsorption.

Q3. Causes of increase phosphorus level.

Ans. Renal failure, hypoparathyroidism, hypervitaminosis D.

Q4. Is there any role of phosphorus in buffer system?

Ans. Yes, phoshphate buffer is main intracellular buffer.

Q5. Write biochemical functions of phosphorus.

Ans. See on last page.

Demonstration

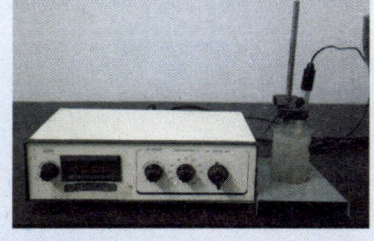
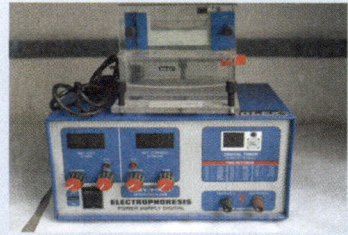

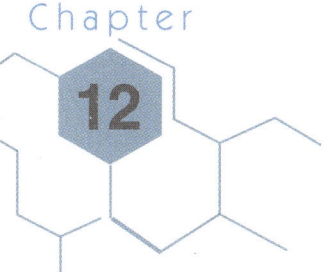
pH Meter

INTRODUCTION

pH meter is an instrument used to determine the pH of a solution.

Principle: pH meter is based on the principle of measurement of ECF (electromotive force), generated between two electrode. This force occurs due to difference in hydrogen ion concentration.

When metal plate kept in a solution of its own salt, it loses ions into the solution and it becomes negatively charged.

- Metal plate—negatively charged (zinc).
- Solution—positively charged (zinc sulfate).

If two different metal plate (electrode) are used in which one act as reference electrode (known potential) and other electrode whose potential we want to measure.

Reference Electrode

- Standard hydrogen electrode.
- Calomel electrode.
- Glass electrode.
- Combined electrode.

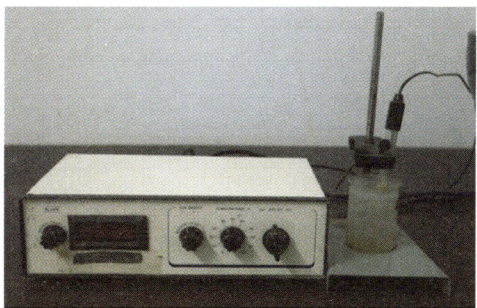

Fig. 12.1: pH meter

Procedure

1. Adjust temperature by knob in pH meter.
2. First of all wash electrode with water, wipe with soft tissue paper.
3. Take various standard buffer for pH 4, 7, 9.
4. Calibrate the instruments with 7 pH, then 4 and 9, 10.
5. Then dip unknown solution and read pH.
6. After this wash it again and dip into DW.

Precautions

1. Always wash electrode after use, dip into DW.
2. Followed any specific guideline provided by instrument manual.
3. Temperature correction is also required for assessment of pH.

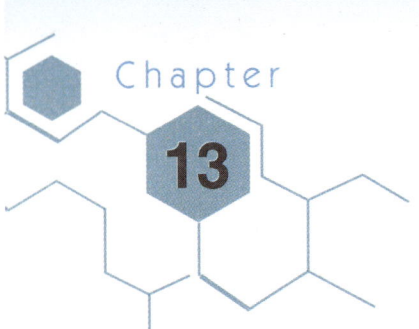

Chromatography

DEFINITION

This technique is used for the separation of closely related compounds, present in a mixture solution like carbohydrates, lipid, amino acids, vitamins, etc. The term was given by Mikhail Tswett.

Principle: Separation of mixture by chromatography depends on Stationary and Mobile phase. There is movement of solute mixture in Mobile phase, which move on Stationary phase. This interaction, results in separation of compounds.

Migration of substance is measured as R_f (ratio of front) value

$$R_f = \frac{\text{Distance travelled by substance (solute)}}{\text{Distance travelled by solvent}}$$

Classification

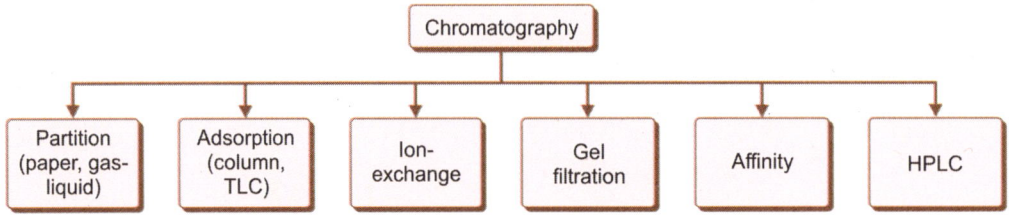

Paper Chromatography

Aim: Separation of individual amino acids from a mixture.

Requirements

- Lead pencil.
- Filter paper strip, (Whatman no 1).
- Amino acid mixture (tyrosine, aspartic acid, alanine) (Fig. 13.2).
- Solvent mixture (Butanol: Acetic acid: DW, 12 : 3 : 5).
- Chromatography chamber (Fig. 13.1).
- Capillary tube, pipette, oven, dryer.
- Ninhydrin.

Procedure

- Make 2% solution of amino acid mixture (0.2 gm in 100 ml).
- Cover beaker with aluminum foil to prevent it from oxidation and protection from direct sunlight and air.
- Make buffer solution 12 : 3 : 5.
- Take A clean TLC chamber.
- Take paper and mark two line-one horizontal, one vertical.

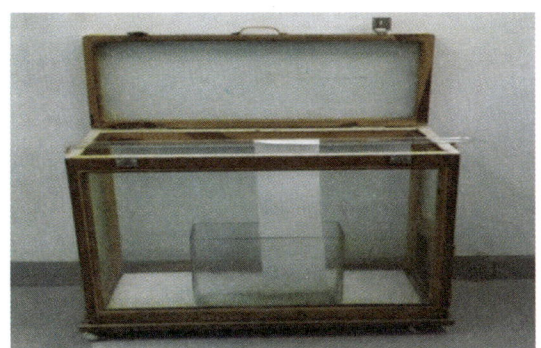

Fig. 13.1: Chromatography chamber

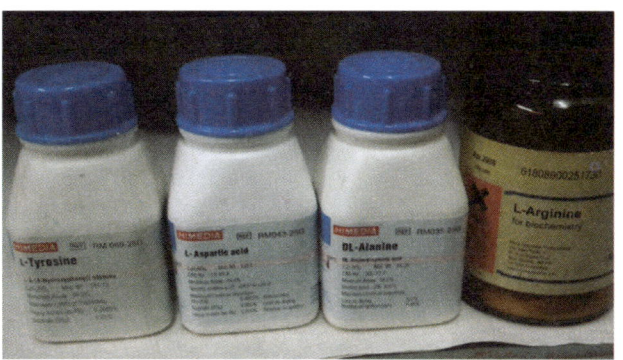

Fig. 13.2: Amino acids for chromatography

- Mark three point on horizontal line.
- With the help of capillary put first solution on Ist mark.
- Marked dot on horizontal line.
- Then dry it with the help of dryer.
- Repeat it with more solutions.
- Keep buffer solution in TLC chamber.
- Put TLC paper into the chamber along the side wall such that the horizontal line get completely emerged into the solution.
- Then wait for 40 minutes for allowing into stand.
- After 40 minutes take paper out of chamber, and dry.
- Dry for 20 minutes in oven, or help of dryer.
- After that stain will appear on the paper (Fig. 13.3).
- Spry ninhydrin on the stain.
- Mark it with lead pencil.
- Measure the distance from starting of horizontal line to the end point and also measure horizontal-vertical line.
- Calculate Rf value.
- According this substance can be found out.

Result

Calculate R_f value

$$R_f = \frac{\text{Distance travelled by substance}}{\text{Distance travelled by solvent}}$$

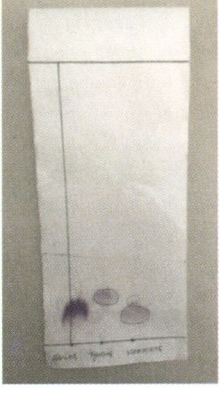

Fig. 13.3: Paper chromatography of amino acids

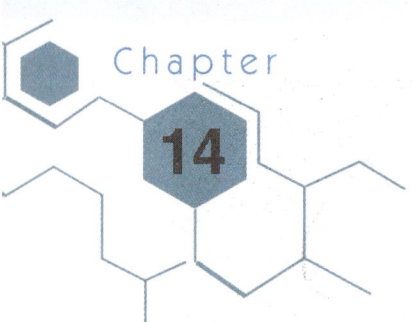

Electrophoresis

DEFINITION

It is a technique widely used for the separation of biological molecules like plasma proteins, lipoproteins, immunoglobulin, etc.

Principle: When charged particles are subjected to electric field they move towards the opposite poles, negatively charged particles move towards the anode and positively charged particle move towards the cathode.

For example, in alkaline medium proteins are negatively charged, when electric field is applied they move towards the anode.

Migration of particles in electric current depends on following factors:

1. Charge on ions.
2. Strength of electric current.
3. Size and shape of the charge particles.
4. Temperature.
5. Ionic strength buffer.
6. Support medium properties.

Procedure

- Sample is applied on a support media.
- The medium is then placed in a buffer solution, filled in electrophoresis chamber.
- Electric current is passed through the media to carry out electrophoresis.
- Support medium is removed and stained to visualize the separated bands.

Types of Electrophoresis

Free electrophoresis	Zone electrophoresis
It is of two types:	**It has following types:**
1. Microelectrophoresis	1. Paper
2. Moving boundary electrophoresis	2. Cellulose acetate
Out dated, mostly used for non-biological experiments	3. Capillary
	4. Gel: Further classified into:
	a. Agarose gel
	b. SDS-PAGE
	c. PFGE
	d. Two dimensional

Paper electrophoresis: Support medium is a filter paper having adsorptive capacity and uniform pore size. Filter paper is moistened with buffer and ends of the strip are immersed into buffer reservoirs containing the electrodes.

Cellulose acetate electrophoresis: It is a modified version of paper electrophoresis, where instead of filter paper, cellulose acetate membrane is used.

Capillary electrophoresis: Capillarity of narrow bore tube is employed to separate the samples based on their size: charge ratio.

Gel electrophoresis: Gel is used as a support media for the separation of DNA, RNA and proteins under the influence of electric current. It is the most commonly used technique.

Type of gel electrophoresis

Agarose gel	Agarose gel
	Used for separation of nucleic acid
SDS- sodium dodecyl sulfate polyacrylamide gel electrophoresis	Used to separate proteins SDS dissociates proteins into individual polypeptide subunit and gives a uniform negative charge
Pulse field gel electrophoresis	Agarose/polyacrylamide gel molecules are induced to migrate through the gel under a static electric field. DNA, under the influence of electric field elongate and align themselves with the field
Two-dimensional electrophoresis	Used to purify protein mixture ampholyte solution is incorporated into the gel. A stable pH gradient is established in the gel after application of electric field. This is followed by SDS-PAGE

Aim: To perform agarose gel electrophoresis to separate mixture of protein/nucleic acid.

Principle: Molecules are separated based on molecular size. Agarose gel acts as a sieve. Larger and bulky molecules stay behind whereas the smaller molecules move faster and quickly towards their respective electrodes.

Instruments required:

1. Electrophoretic chamber (Fig. 14.1).
2. Power supply.
3. Trans-illuminator, to visualize the DNA in gel.
4. Agarose gel support media.
5. Buffer: TAE buffer or tris acetate EDTA (Fig. 14.2).
6. Ethidium bromide dye to stain the DNA.

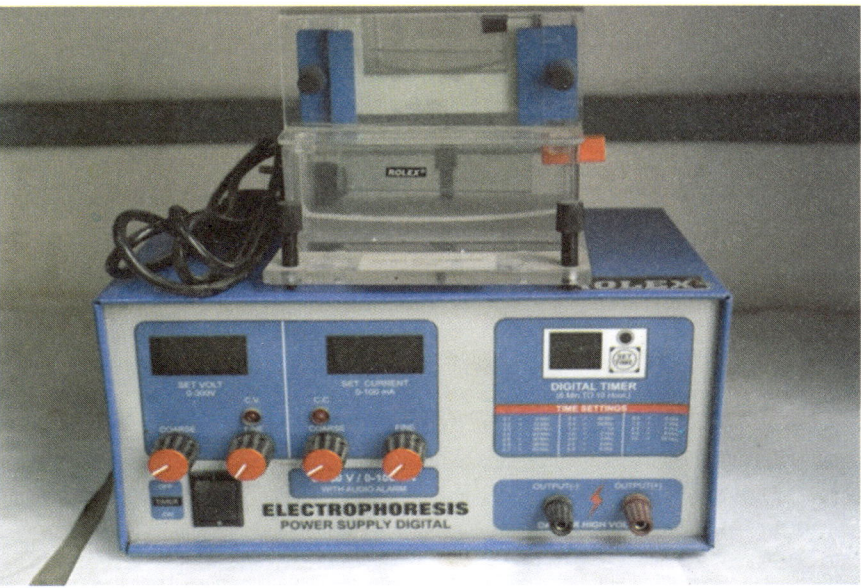

Fig. 14.1: Electrophoretic chamber and power supply

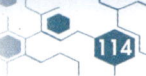

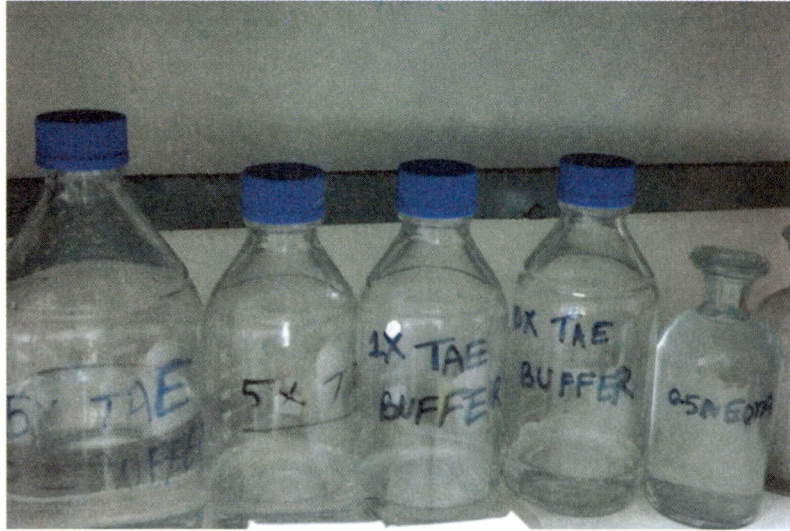

Fig. 14.2: Reagents required for electrophoresis

Procedure

1. *Formation of agarose gel*: Dry agarose gel powder is mixed with electrophoresis buffer to the desired concentration and heated till it completely melts.
2. Ethidium bromide 0.5 mg/ml is added at this point.
3. After cooling at 60°C it is added into the casting tray containing sample comb and allowed to solidify at room temperature. Once the gel is dry sample comb is removed.
4. The gel is removed and placed in electrophoretic chamber and covered with buffer.
5. Sample containing the mixture of DNA and buffer is applied on sample well.
6. Lid and power leads are placed on the apparatus and current is applied.
7. Current flow is confirmed by the presence of bubbles.
8. DNA being negatively charged move towards the positive electrode.
9. Ethidium bromide gets incorporated into the DNA. Once separation has occurred the fragments of DNA can be visualized in a UV trans-illuminator.

Preparation of Buffer

Tris buffer: 3 gm tris, 0.39 gm EDTA and 0.23 gm boric acid are dissolved in 250 ml distilled water.

1% agarose: 0.1 gm of dry agarose powder is dissolved in 10 ml tris buffer and boiled till it is completely dissolved.

DNA Extraction

Procedure of DNA extraction.

Step 1: Source of DNA

a. Cell culture up to 5×10^6 cells should be present.
b. Tissue up to 25 mg.
c. Blood/serum up to 200 µl.

Step 2: Cell lysis—to Remove Proteins, Lipids and RNA

a. Lipids are removed with the help of detergents/surfactants.
b. Proteins are removed with the help of enzyme proteinase.
c. RNA is removed with help of RNAase.

Cell debris consisting of amino acids, lipids, RNAs are clumped together by treating with saline. Centrifugation removes clumped cell debris from DNA.

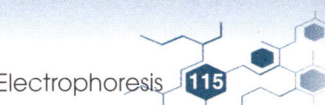

Step 3: DNA Purification

There are three methods of DNA purification:

a. **Ethanol precipitation:** DNA being insoluble in ethanol aggregates in it and form pellets on centrifugation.

b. **Phenol:** Chloroform extraction—protein is denatured by phenol and it remains in the organic phase. DNA being insoluble in phenol stays in the aqueous phase. DNA is separated from aqueous phase and treated with chloroform to remove phenol residue.

c. **Minicolumn purification:** Column chromatography which relies on the principle, nucleic acid binds with solid phase depending on pH and salt concentration of the solution.

Once the DNA is removed it is kept in alkaline buffer like TE buffer or ultra pure water.

Protein Electrophoresis Interpretation

Normal serum on electrophoresis gets separated into 5 bands

Albumin	55–60%
α1 globulin	3–4%
α2 globulin	5–10%
β globulin	9–10%
γ globulin	10–20%

Pathological conditions identified on serum protein electrophoresis

1. Nephrotic syndrome	Loss of albumin in urine, albumin band will reduce
2. Liver cirrhosis	Albumin is not synthesized Albumin band will reduce with wide β globulin band
3. Chronic infection	γ globulin increases
4. Multiple myeloma	A sharp spike is seen in γ globulin, called M-band

Miscellaneous

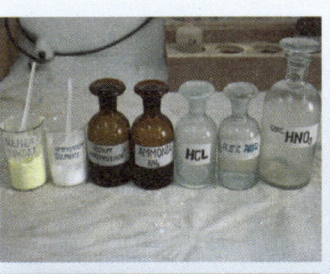
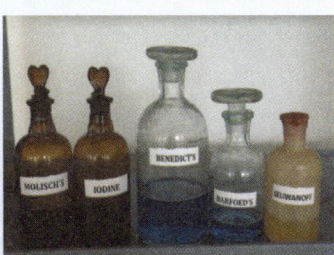
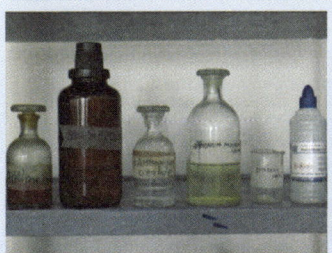
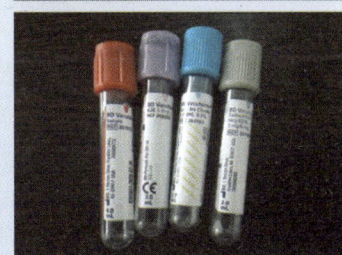

Body Fluids

Collection, prevention and analysis of body fluid

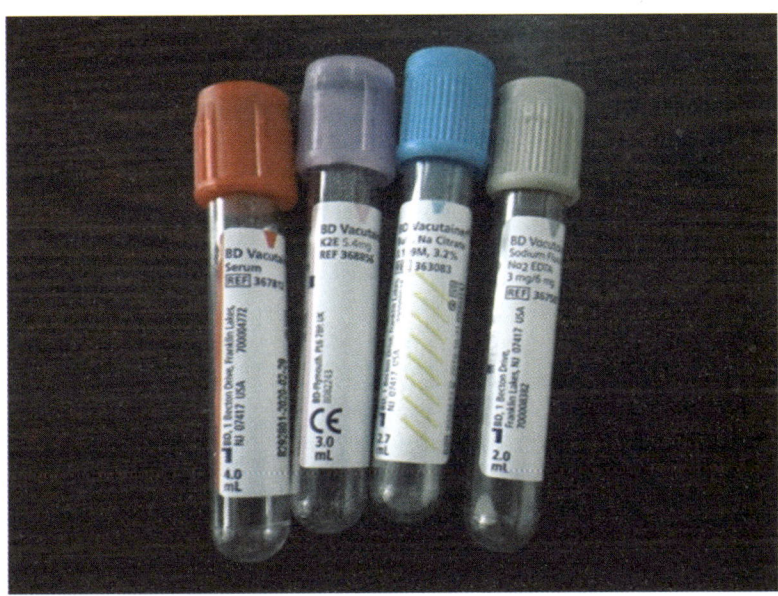

Fig. 15.1: Various vials used for collection

Types of Fluid
- Milk
- CSF (cerebrospinal fluid)
- AF (ascites fluid)
- PF (pleural fluid)
- Amniotic fluid
- Synovial fluid
- Pericardial fluid.

CSF: Collection of sample by lumbar puncture.
- Fluid is collected in 3 to 4 plain tubes.
- CSF in first tube act as a reserve sample.
- Biochemistry and immunological tests are performed on second tube.
- Culture and other tests related to microbiology are performed on third test tube.
- Tests related to hematology are performed on forth test tube.

   If CSF fluid is available in only three test tubes then, biochemistry, immunology and hematology, tests related to all three are performed on third test tube.

RBC's are normally absent in CSF, but it can be present in case of traumatic tap or subarachnoid hemorrhage, to differentiate between the two conditions RBC count is performed on first tube and third/fourth tube:

In case of traumatic tap, RBC's will be present in only in tube since first tube is filled first.

In case of subarachnoid hemorrhage RBC's will be present in both tubes 1 and 3/4

CSF findings in various pathological conditions

	Normal	Tuberculosis meningitis	Bacterial meningitis	Subarachnoid hemorrhage	Brain tumor
Color and appearance	Clear and colorless	Opalescent and Cob web formed on standing, yellow	Turbid	Blood color	Clear and colorless
Total cell count	0–5	Increased	Markedly increase	RBC's present	No change
Protein	15–45 mg/dl	Increased	Markedly increase	Increased	Increased
Glucose	45–85 mg/dl	Low	Markedly low	Increased	Low

Pleural Fluid

Collection done in 4 mL in lavender top spray coated EDTA tube or dark green top sodium heparin tube.

Biochemical Analysis

- Protein 0–2 gm/dl, sugar 50–70 mg/dl, Cl 95–108 mEqµl/L.
- ADA (adenosine deaminase estimation in pleural fluid is done) 0–10 normal, >10 infection.

AF (Ascites Fluid)

- Sample required > 25 Ml.
- Protein 0–2 gm/dl, sugar 50–70 mg/dl , Cl 95–108 mEq/L, SAAG (serum albumin—ascites albumin).

Synovial Fluid for Crystal

Preferred sample—4 ml dark green top sodium heparin tube, not plasma seperated tube (PST).

Also acceptable

- Sterile container (no additive).
- Red top tube.
- Lavender top spray coated EDTA tube.

  Synovial fluid for glucose and protein: 0.5 ml in gold top SST or light green (mint) top PST tube.

  Dialysate: 3–5 mL in lavender top spray coated EDTA tube.

Precautions

- Always indicate priority of test orders on the requisition.
- Pleural fluid pH must be collected in a blood gas syringe.
- Do not send other fluids in syringes (with or without needles attached).
- All body fluids must be taken to the laboratory immediately after collection. Hand the specimen directly to the laboratory personnel (do not leave on counter).

Reagents Preparation

Reagents for Carbohydrates Tests

Reagents	Method of preparation
1. Molisch's reagent	1 gm of α naphthol in 100 ml of ethanol
2. Benedict's reagent	A. 17 gm of sodium citrate and 10 gm of sodium carbonate in 90 ml of distilled water
	B. 1.73 gm of copper sulfate in 10 ml of distilled water
3. Barfoed's reagent	6.6 gm copper acetate and 0.9 ml of glacial acetate in 100 ml of distilled water
4. Seliwanoff's reagent	50 mg resorcinol in 100 ml of 12% HCl
5. 12% HCl	12 ml of HCl in 88 ml of distilled water
6. Iodine solution	1.27 gm iodine and 3 gm of potassium iodide in 100 of distilled water

Reagents for Test of Lipids

Reagents	Method of preparation
1. Emulsification sodium carbonate 0.5%	0.5 gm sodium carbonate in 100 ml of distilled water
2. Saponification	
a. KOH/NaOH (10%)	10 ml (KOH/NaOH) in 90 ml of distilled water
b. $CaCl_2$ (5%)	5 gm $CaCl_2$ in 100 ml of ditilled water
3. Dustan test 0.5% boric solution	0.5 gm of boric powder in 100 ml of distilled water
4. Hubel's iodine	26 gm of iodine and 30 gm of $HgCl_2$ in 1000 ml of ethanol

Reagents for Tests of Proteins

Reagents	Method of preparation
1. Biuret test	10% NaOH—10 gm NaOH in 100 ml DW
	0.5% copper sulfate—0.5 gm copper sulfate in 100 ml DW
2. Ninhydrin reagent (2%)	2 gm ninhydrin in 100 ml DW
3. Xanthoproteic test	40 gm NaOH in 100 ml DW
4. 40% NaOH	
5. Millon's reagent	10 gm mercuric sulfate in 50 ml DW and 10 ml conc H_2SO_4, make final volume 100 ml with DW
6. Sodium nitrate 1%	1 gm in 100 ml of DW
7. Hopkin cole's	40% formaline reagent 1 ml formaline in 500 ml DW
8. Sakaguchi reagent	Molisch's reagent, sodium hypobromite-1 ml bromine in 100 ml of 10% NaOH
	10% NaOH is 10 gm NaOH in 100 ml DW
9. 2% lead acetate	2 gm lead acetate in 100 ml DW
10. Esbach's reagent	5 gm picric acid and 10 gm citric acid in 500 ml DW

Reagents for Normal Urine

Reagents for uric acid	0.1 N AgNO₃ 1.7 GM AgNO₃ in 100 ml DW
Reagents for phosphate	Conc nitric acid 25 gm ammonium molybdate + 200 ml DW + 300 ml 10 N H_2SO_4

How to form Normal and Molar Solution

$M_1V_1 = M_2V_2$ (number of solute per mole) W/V

$N_1V_1 = N_2V_2$

5M H_2SO_4 (98%)

$M_1V_1 = M_2V_2$

$5 \times 1000 = 18.4 \times V_2$

5000/18.4

271 ml

10 N H_2SO_4 (98%)

$M_1 = 10N = 5M$

$M_1V_1 = M_2V_2$

$5 \times 1000 = 18.4 \times V_2$

$V_2 = 5000/18.4$

271.7 ml

9N H_2SO_4 (98%)

$9 \times 1000 = 36.8 \times V_2$

$9000/36.8 = V_2$

244.56 ml

.25 N HCL (36%)

$.25 \times 1000 = 11.65 \times V_2$

$V_2 = 250/11.65$

21.45 ml

N/5 NaOH

$N_1 = N/5, N_2 = 19.4, V_1 = 1000$

N/5 × 1000/19.4

200/19.4 = 10.30 gm.

Note: Add required volume of DW to make up to 1000 ml of solution.

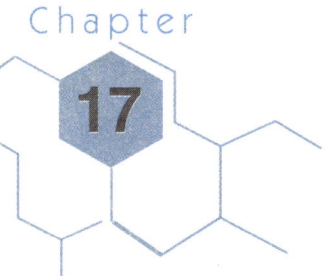
Biological Waste Disposal

Any material containing infectious material is called biomedical waste. Biological waste is segregated into appropriately colored plastic bags.

I. Red category: Recyclable infected waste.

1. Tubes
2. Bottles
3. Soiled gloves
4. Urine bags
5. Syringes
6. IV sets
7. ET tubes
8. All medical plastic equipment.

Disposed by: Autoclaving/microwaving, hydroclaving followed by shredding or mutilation or combination (Fig. 17.1).

II. Blue category: Recyclable waste (glassware)

1. Broken glass
2. Contaminated glass
3. Medicine vials
4. Ampoules
5. Metallic body parts.

Disposed by: Disinfection by sodium hypochlorite treatment or through autoclaving, microwaving, hydroclaving (Fig. 17.2).

III. White category: Infected sharp waste

1. Needles
2. Blades
3. Scalpels
4. Burnt needle
5. Syringes with fixed needles
6. All medical used metallic sharps.

Disposed by: Autoclaving or dry heat, sterilization, followed by shredding, mutilation or combination (Fig. 17.3).

IV. Yellow category: Waste contaminated with blood body fluid and infected cytotoxic waste.

1. Discarded medicine
2. Human anatomical waste

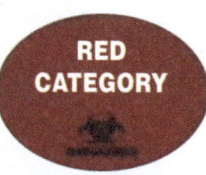

Recyclable infected waste (plastic)
- Tubes
- Bottles (plastic)
- Gloves even soiled
- Urine bags
- Syringes (without needles)
- IV sets
- ET tubes
- All medical plastic equipment

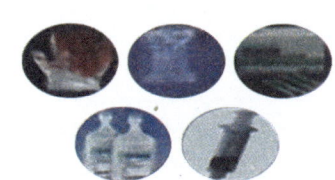

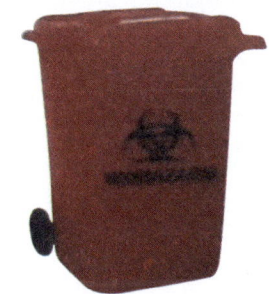

Fig. 17.1: Autoclaving/microwaving, hydroclaving followed by shredding or multilation or combination

BLUE CATEGORY

Recyclable waste (glassware)
• Broken glass
• Contaminated glass
• Medicine vials
• Ampoules
• Metallic body implants

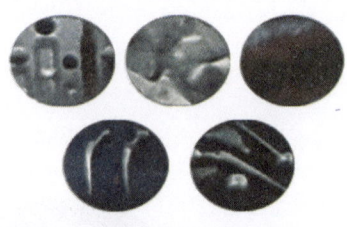

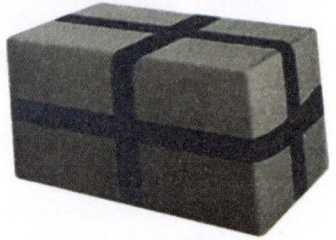

Fig. 17.2: Disinfection by soldium hypochlorite treatment of through autoclaving, microwaving, hydroclaving

WHITE CATEGORY

Infected sharp waste (sharp container: Puncture proof, leak proof, temper proof, translucent)
• Needles
• Blades
• Scalpels
• Burnt needles
• Syrings with fixed needles
• All medical used metallic sharps

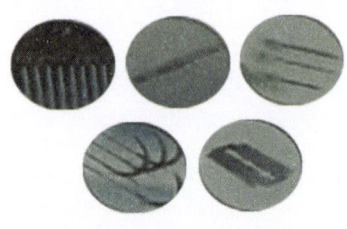

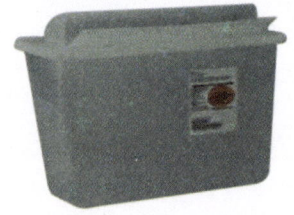

Fig. 17.3: Autoclaving or dry heat, sterilization, followed by shredding, mutilation or combination

3. Soiled linen and bedding/mattresses

4. Soiled waste

5. Animal anatomical waste

6. Blood bags

7. Expired medicines

8. Microbiology, clinical and laboratory waste (after pretreatment)

9. Cytotoxic drugs

10. Items contaminated with cytotoxic drugs

11. Infected with cytotoxic secretions.

Disposed by: Incineration or plasma pyrolysis or deep burial (Fig. 17.4).

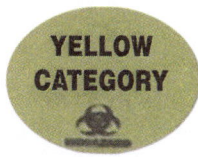

Waste contaminated with blood body fluid and infected cytotoxic waste
- Discarded medicine
- Human anatomical waste
- Soiled linen and beddings/ mattresses
- Soiled waste
- Blood bags
- Expired medicines
- Microbiology, clinical and laboratory waste (after pretreatment)
- Cytotoxic drugs
- Items contaminated with cytotoxic drugs
- Infected with cytotoxic secretions

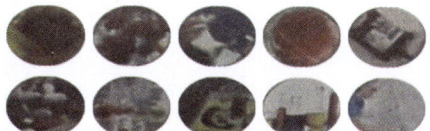

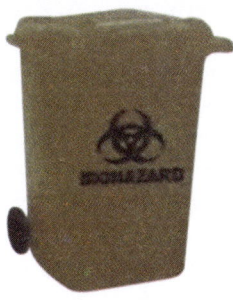

Fig. 17.4: Management incineration or plasma pyrolysis or deep burial

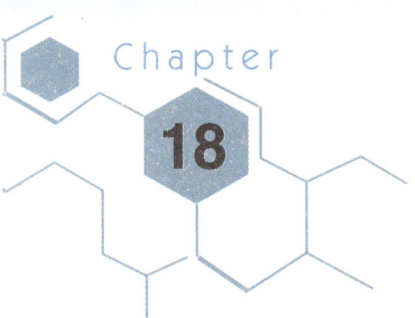

Blood Gas Analyzer

INTRODUCTION

Measurement of blood gases, pH and electrolytes, metabolite, bicarbonate concentration by blood gas analyzer (Fig. 18.1).

Principle: pH, PCO_2, PO_2 can be directly measured by analyzer. Generation of potential difference between two electrodes is responsible for measurement of pH, PCO_2 and PO_2. Hb is measured in percentage saturation. Bicarbonate concentration calculated by Handerson–Hasselbach equation. For the measurement of electrolytes Na^+, K^+, Ca^{++}, Cl^-, Li^+ ion selective electrode (ISE) method is used.

Sample: Arterial heparinised whole blood sample, volume 70–100 µl.

Procedure: As per the manual provided with instrument.

Precaution

- Arterial blood sample should be used.
- Blood sample should not be clotted.
- Analyze the sample as soon as possible within half an hour.
- Instrument should be washed after or between uses of samples.

Clinical Applications

- Acid-base disorders.
- Critical care patients.
- Burn cases.

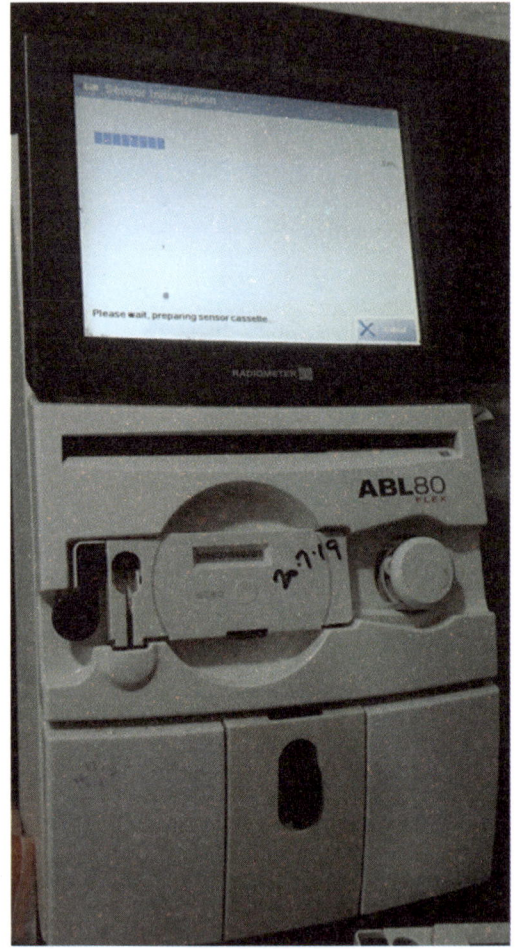

Fig. 18.1